Magic, Myth and Medicine

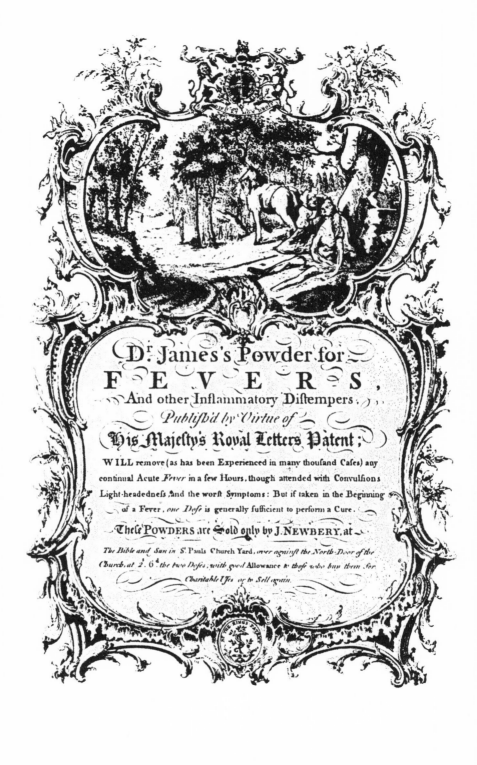

Magic, Myth and Medicine

JOHN CAMP

Taplinger Publishing Company
NEW YORK

First Published in the United States in 1974 by
TAPLINGER PUBLISHING CO., INC.
New York, New York

Published simultaneously in the Dominion of Canada by
Burns & MacEachern, Ltd., Toronto

Library of Congress Catalog Card Number: 73-18793

ISBN 0-8008-5046-7

CONTENTS

ILLUSTRATIONS

Text figures

Magic, Myth and Medicine

1

The Instinct for Survival

THE instinct for survival shows itself in many ways in man and animals. Its most basic and primitive form is the instinct to flee from danger, or, if this is impossible, to turn and face the aggressor. But the dangers that threaten living things cannot always be seen and recognized. They appear in many insidious ways. Life itself is doomed from the outset, and the process of ageing, beginning at birth, exerts its influence until it is finally triumphant.

Since man first appeared on earth illness has taken its toll, accelerating the ageing process and bringing life to an end before its natural term. Even the fossilized skeletons of dinosaurs 200 million years old display evidence of rheumatism and arthritis. Human Stone Age skeletons bear witness to fractured bones and their subsequent healing and, from ancient times, skulls have been found showing unmistakable signs of trepanning, the operation in which the skull is bored to relieve pressure on the brain.

For early man, in his cave or mud hut, illness was known and feared. Even non-fatal diseases could be a danger, by reducing man's capacity to hunt or fight, and so endangering his ability to survive. The ways in which man tried to circumvent disaster took many forms and provide the basis of the folklore and superstition surrounding preventive medicine that survives today. Before he could try to combat illness man needed to recognize some of the causative factors involved. Some explanation was needed, some reason given, why human beings were afflicted in so many ways. Why did one man's wounds heal and another's not? Why did some children die and others live? Why was one hunting expedition a success and another a calamity? For primitive man there was only one answer—an unknown and all-powerful force was at work shaping men's lives and expressing pleasure or displeasure at their actions.

Every culture has found it necessary to believe in some form of divine providence. How else could one explain the greatest works of Nature, the ebb and flow of the tides, the rising and setting of the sun, the coming and going of the seasons? If the gods could so control the elements it was logical to attribute to them the disasters that they so often caused. The result was a primitive but organized response to such happenings. Misfortunes, it was held, came about through the breaking of laws which incurred the anger of the gods. Atonement could be made only by conciliation.

During thousands of years a pattern of causative factors has evolved held to be responsible for illness. They survive today in the beliefs of primitive peoples the world over, and may be broadly defined as follows:

1. Sorcery or witchcraft
2. The breaking of taboos
3. The intrusion of disease-objects
4. The action of disease-spirits
5. Loss of soul.

The relative importance of these factors varies widely from one culture to another. For example sorcery, witchcraft and the breaking of taboos is most prevalent in the continent of Africa, while loss of "soul" is held to be the chief reason for calamity among the North American Eskimos and the peoples of Siam, Mexico and China. It is this belief that the soul of man can be extracted, and removed in the form of an image, that accounts for the persistent antagonism of these peoples to attempts to draw or photograph them. The soul, their most treasured possession, has been captured by the camera or artist and misfortune will inevitably result.

From earliest times there were individual men who seemed to have special powers and be in particular *rapport* with the deities. These were the wise—or "witch"—men who acted as a channel of communication between their fellows and the gods they worshipped. As a combination of magician, doctor and priest they enjoyed immense status and were sometimes treated as royalty. In some civilizations the situation was reversed, and kingship itself was held to include magical powers, such as healing.

Both Tacitus and Suetonius tell how the Roman Emperor Vespasian made apparently miraculous cures with his touch. In Britain the first King known to claim such powers was Edward the Confessor, who "touched" for scrofula in 1058. But in most cultures, even if the witch-doctor did not attain royal status, he became a powerful and feared figure. Not only was he expected to cure illness but also to predict the future, speak with the dead and, perhaps most important of all, to ensure the victory of his tribe in battle and to bring calamity upon the enemy. In his role as a prophet the witch-doctor took a strong interest in practical matters. For example, when should the tribe sow crops, or mount an attack on a neighbouring tribe? He invoked the aid of astrology to determine the presence of good or evil forces at work in his community.

But in the field of medicine and healing he had rather more practical means at his disposal. All around him, in the fields and forests, lay the vast *herbarium* of plant life. He knew that sick animals had recourse to the curative power of various plants. But it was not enough just to use these plants for their therapeutic properties. For illness was an affliction brought about by offending the gods, and cures could only be made by placating the gods. The art of curing was hedged about with magic and taboo. For example, the use of peonies as a cure for epilepsy was nullified if one looked at a woodpecker while picking the flower, and the unlucky victim would probably go blind. Taboos such as these were the stock-in-trade of witch-doctors, and medicine-men.

Among the taboos connected with illness the "uncleanness" of a woman during menstruation or pregnancy is by far the commonest. From Alaska to Africa, Europe to Australia, taboos are found forbidding association with, or even touching, a woman during childbirth or while having a menstrual flow. Among the American Indians a young girl who showed the first signs of menstruation was an object of dread. She was hidden from public gaze, and forbidden to eat the flesh of venison or any hunted animal in case she insulted the species and brought bad luck to those who hunted it. Sir James Frazer (*The Golden Bough*) tells how an aboriginal of Australia found that his wife had menstruated on his blanket. He immediately killed her, and himself died of terror within a fortnight. In some areas a woman is shut off from all contact with others for three weeks after childbirth and food is handed to her on a stick to avoid contagion. Most dangerous of all is the result of a hidden miscarriage, for the production of blood which does not "congeal" into a new human being is taken as proof that the woman has committed great sins. The Bantu believe that the blood of such a woman is infectious not only to her community but to the country as a whole. An amazing machinery of prophylaxis against the spread of the infection is carried out reaching to the borders of the country and embracing every other community within it. In the same way strenuous efforts are made to avoid the import of disease-objects to a community. When strangers arrive precautions are taken to placate the gods against the diseases, and so the sins, of the new arrivals. When tribesmen return to their native village complex purification processes are used by the medicine-man or witch-doctor, in case they have brought back disease by contact or in a trophy from the enemy.

The number of taboos among primitive peoples is legion, and embraces virtually every action and almost every object. There is said to be great danger in eating or drinking, for when the mouth is open malignant spirits can easily enter the body, or the soul escape. In either case illness or death will follow. The danger is considered so great in some societies that to protect the king from possible contagion from his subjects it is forbidden to watch him eat or drink. In some African tribes if a dog or other animal strays into the compound where the king is drinking, it is instantly put to death by the knife. One case is recorded where the twelve-year-old son of the tribal chief was hacked to death when he unwittingly came upon his father enjoying a meal.

Parallel with man's ancient belief in the gods is his belief in an "inner man" or soul. In most instances it is thought to exist as a replica in the shape of man himself, and lives in various parts of the body. The Eskimos believe the soul is a tiny figure located in the head. Normally it stands erect, but if for any reason it falls madness will follow. Most common is the belief that the soul leaves the body during illness and in sleep. Medicine-men in many parts of the world devise ways of closing every orifice of the body during illness to avoid the escape of the soul, and death. A common object found in the *armamentarium* of witch-doctors is a small bottle or flask in which the soul can be trapped and returned again to its rightful owner. In European countries it is more common to find the belief that the escaping soul takes the form of a small animal, often a mouse, and in remote areas it is still a common practice to close the mouth of a sleeping child in case his soul should escape. Some folk believe that during sleep the soul is always absent. They believe it would be fatal to awaken a sleeping person, as the soul may not have time to return, and a fatal illness or other calamity will follow. Some Pacific islanders believe that in illness the soul of the sick man leaves to join the souls of those dead and buried. The villagers leave the patient's bedside and walk to the burial-ground, where they play flutes and other wind instruments imploring the soul to return, and so restore the victim to health. In some cultures a man's shadow is said to be his soul, and may be contaminated by contact with the dead or dying. At a funeral, therefore, the shadow of a mourner or close relative must never fall on anyone watching, or the fate of the dead person will overtake the watcher.

A curious belief still exists in some parts of Greece and Romania, associating the soul with the future health of those who are to live in a new building. The soul is sometimes represented by a cock or a sheep, and the animal is killed and its blood poured into the foundations. In Romania the custom has rather more sinister implications, for it is only the soul of a man that can bring good health to the future inhabitants of the house, and if a man loses his soul he will die. The builder chooses a victim, tries to measure the length of his shadow without being seen and buries the rule under the foundation stone. The unsuspecting victim goes cheerfully on his way, having unknowingly brought health and prosperity to a houseful of strangers, but invited death to claim him within a year! For this reason it is common practice in Greece and Romania to warn strangers passing a new building with the cry—"Watch out for your soul!"—though the results of this curious brand of pilfering are no longer held to be fatal.

Almost certainly fatal, it was believed in India and ancient Greece, was to look at one's reflection in water. The soul was in the reflection and the water spirits could easily pull it below the surface, bringing illness and death. This is why, in some communities, mirrors are never left uncovered in a sick person's room in case he should see his reflection and his soul escape. By the same token, the patient is never allowed to sleep, for his soul, absent in sleep, may represent a danger to the sufferer by delaying its return and so hastening death.

In these and many other ways people the world over take precautions against illness. There seems little logic in most of the methods used, though many customs contain some scientific elements of which the participants are totally unaware. Such is the custom observed in the New Hebrides of burying all left-over food in case it should be found by enemies and magic wrought with it. In fact, the custom ensures that harmful bacteria are not disseminated by the rotting flesh. Similarly the taboo found in the South Pacific that food must never be eaten cold is hygienically sound. The reheating will most likely destroy any growing bacteria.

Yet despite these many precautions illness still comes and epidemics strike. It then becomes a question of cure and, for the witch-doctor or medicine-man, of his own survival, for his status depends on the degree of his success. His initial diagnosis was concerned, not primarily with the nature of the disease, but with finding what sin had made the victim vulnerable. First and foremost the patient had to confess, and if he were unable or unwilling to supply the information, then the medicine-man would invoke divine judgement. The sick man is given poison : his death would be proof of his sin. But if he lives it is a sign he is surely innocent and will respond to treatment. Other methods were often used to establish innocence or guilt. The victim might be thrown into a river, or have his affected limb immersed in boiling oil or fire. As late as the eighteenth century such rough-and-ready methods were still in vogue. Two of the most common were the weighing of a suspected witch against the Bible, and "swimming" her across a river.

But the diagnosis of illness was only part of the medicine-man's duties. He also had to prognosticate the probable length of the illness from signs and portents—the unusual flight of birds, for example, or from studying the entrails of slaughtered animals. Only after long

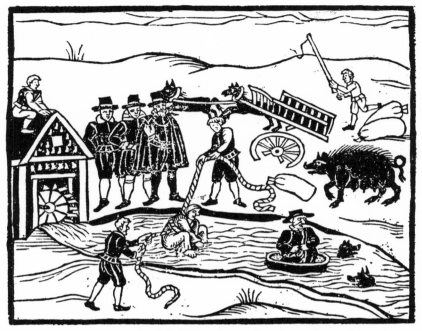

1 Swimming a witch

interrogation of the patient and a detailed study of the likely outcome
of the ailment did the actual process of cure begin.

If the patient admitted to breaking a taboo or committing some
other indiscretion, the first step toward recovery was already taken.
If the victim could point to another person who may have bewitched
him and caused the affliction, then the medicine-man would have a
point on which to focus his therapy.

These activities are normally picturesque and form part of the
window-dressing of the healer in most parts of the world. They
include dancing around the patient, singing, incantations, touching
with healing objects, and making physical contact to try and draw off
the malignant spirits. But in all these methods, many of them highly
bizarre, there is an underlying basis of natural cure. Special and
secret herbs are prepared, instructions are given on washing and diet,
and bleeding and massage are used.

15

In certain primitive peoples there evolved specialists, groups of travelling medicine-men who concerned themselves with specific kinds of disease. The most interesting example is the *shaman*, a medicine-man who concentrates on the cure of mental disorders and who is still found today among Eskimo tribes and in Siberia. The *shaman* must himself have undergone an emotional crisis, preferably at puberty. To effect a cure he must be able to enter an ecstasy or trance at will, drawing the bad spirit out of the afflicted patient and into himself, and by stupendous self-discipline and concentration dispose of it and render it harmless.

In time, certain gods were associated with certain diseases. Just as certain deities were thought to be responsible for fire, flood and other disasters, so others were held responsible for specific illnesses. If propitiated, these gods could alleviate or cure them. Combined with the association of the gods with the known healing properties of plants, together with the growing use of astrology in foretelling the future of the patient, a rich tapestry of medical folklore was woven— part mythology, part medicine, part magic. It is the intricate inter-weaving and the effect on human beliefs which makes folk medicine such a fascinating subject. It is virtually impossible, even today, to separate the strands fully, for the attributes of the gods were slowly translated to human beings, or even to animals and plants. Much of our medical knowledge is based on myths and legends from the dawn of history.

At the time of the ancient Greeks the god of healing was Aesculapius, the son of Apollo and Coronis. Snatched from his mother's funeral pyre, he was brought up by Chiron, a centaur skilled in the hunt and in the arts of healing. The boy showed a special aptitude for the latter. As he grew to manhood Aesculapius became so proficient that he was soon venerated as the god of healing. After his marriage to the goddess Epione, he fathered seven children—two boys and five girls—most of whom were to be associated with medicine and healing, and whose names survive today. Among the daughters was Panacea, goddess of the relief of pain, and Hygiea, goddess of cleanliness. Another daughter, Telesphorus, watched over the convalescent and was shown wearing a hooded cape, the normal dress of those recovering from illness in ancient Greece.

The two sons of Aesculapius, Podalerius and Machaon, inherited their father's skill in healing, and founded the dynasty of healers known as the Aesculepiads. Certain Greek doctors banded themselves together under that name, and indeed there was more myth than medicine in their administrations for many centuries. One of them, Hippocrates, was responsible more than any other for sowing the seeds of medical science and research and bringing healing into the light. His theories and teachings laid the foundations of modern medicine, and the Hippocratic oath, in which this famous physician laid down the duties of the doctor toward his patient, is still taken seriously by the medical profession today.

Hippocrates was one of the first to declare that illness was caused, not by gods or evil spirits, but for biological reasons, and could cure itself by the same means. Five hundred years before (about 3000 B.C.) there had been a curious reversal of the transmutation of a god to a human being in the great Egyptian physician Imhotep. He lived at the court of King Zoser (2980–2900 B.C.) who built the first pyramid. Imhotep was the architect. By reason of his learning and wisdom he came to be associated with the sciences, particularly with medicine, and by the time of the New Kingdom (1600 B.C.) had become the patron of doctors, and elevated to the rank of a god. There is evidence that about this time the Greeks themselves learned of him, and identified him with their own god, Aesculapius. Imhotep was buried at Memphis, capital of the Old Kingdom of Egypt before the provinces were united in the New Kingdom, and the city became a temple of medical learning. Unfortunately, no writings of Imhotep have so far been authenticated. A dozen or so papyri have been found, which shed light on the medicine of the time, and it is possible that at least one is by him.

In 1862 an American amateur Egyptologist called Edwin Smith purchased a great roll of papyri in a bazaar in Luxor, but not until 1922 did new knowledge enable these documents to be translated by James Breasted, and it was 1930 before the whole material was published. In 1876 a German, George Ebers of Leipzig, had also unearthed a papyrus dealing with medical matters, and these various documents, all derived from much older writings, throw dazzling light on Egyptian medicine, which until 1922 was thought to lag far behind the attainment of the ancient Egyptians in other crafts and disciplines. Both the Ebers and the Edwin Smith papyri were written at roughly the same time, or at least reflect part of the sum of medical knowledge in Egypt five thousand years ago.

The Ebers papyrus contains 876 remedies using more than 500 different substances. They include not only a wide variety of plants, but also the deliberate use of unpleasant substances such as human and animal excrement, and a selection of aphrodisiacs including *cantharides* (Spanish Fly) still popular for this purpose. It also lists a variety of "magic" remedies and charms. In this respect it is less scientific than the Edwin Smith papyrus, which concerns itself mainly with surgery, and describes the treatment of forty-eight cases, mostly of wounds. But even the Edwin Smith papyrus has an optimistic note, and a magical prescription and incantation is given "for the changing of an old man into a youth of twenty years."

Largely owing to the influence of Hippocrates, ancient Greece is commonly held to be the cradle of medicine. But this is not so. From the seventh century B.C. the Greeks came to Egypt to study medicine and other arts, and eventaully surpassed their masters. But, in the words of the great German medical historian, Dr. Kurt Pollack, "Who will dare to take down Hippocrates from his pedestal as the father of medicine and set up Imhotep in his place?"

Contemporary with the Greek and Egyptian civilizations medical progress was being made in India during the Vedic Epoch, in Persia, and particularly in China. According to legend the Chinese Emperor Shen-nung (2800 B.C.) not only discovered the healing properties of plants, but had his stomach wall removed and replaced with glass so that he could examine the action of the plants inside him! But it was another Emperor, Huang-Ti (2600 B.C.), who was the true founder of Chinese medicine and whose teaching has been written down in a book called *The Theory of Internal Disease* which is still in use today.

It is clear that the study of medicine had been growing in different cultures for three thousand years before the coming of Christ. It is all the more difficult, then, to understand the hostility of the early Christian Church to medicine and healing. This hostility was based on the doctrine of the vanity of earthly happiness, and the need to prepare for the bliss of the next world. Secondly, just as the ancients believed their gods to be responsible for disease, so the Christians believed that God alone had the power of healing. To them it was blasphemy to seek to divert the divine will. The miraculous cures of Jesus underlined this, already expressed in the Old Testament (*Exodus* 15 : 26) when God said to Moses ". . . I will put none of these diseases upon thee, which I have brought on the Egyptians, for I am the lord that healeth thee." Even if not actively hostile towards doctors, the Bible is frequently sceptical, as witness *Ecclesiasticus* 38 : 12–15 : "He who sins before his maker, may he fall into the care of a physician."

Job, wrestling with his many afflictions, had an understandable scepticism where doctors were concerned. He called them "forgers of lies and physicians of no value." The hostility of the early Church to medicine and healing seems, today, at odds with the Christian precepts of charity and compassion. But the terrible God of the Old Testament did not change overnight, with the coming of Christianity, to the more merciful yet more remote God of the Christian era. Hostility and scepticism to medical advance lingered on for centuries, and is with us yet. The Victorian resistance to the use of anaesthesia in childbirth may have been partly due to medical considerations by doctors, but for the average woman it was based far more on the feeling that it was "sinful" to interfere with a natural and so divinely-arranged function.

Medical progress has been shackled by many factors in its long history. For fifteen hundred years at least after Christ progress was retarded by the Humoral Theory, in which all ills were attributed to the malfunction of one of the four "humours" of which the body was said to be composed—black bile, yellow bile, blood and phlegm. In the light of this muddled thinking, and the notorious inability of doctors to agree among themselves, it is easy to see why the common man clung to his ancient beliefs and superstitions. Even doctors were guilty of perpetuating many myths and superstitions. In a book written as late as 1900 by an American gynaecologist, Dr. Emma Angell Drake, the author seriously advises expectant mothers to "look at beautiful pictures, study perfect pieces of statuary and forbid as far as possible the contemplation of unsightly and imperfect models." This, she contends, will ensure "beautiful, vigorous children," and as proof of this, points out how many Italian children bear a resemblance to Jesus Christ as the result of their mothers constantly looking at the religious pictures and statues found in Roman Catholic homes! Many beliefs such as these, their roots lost in antiquity, still flourish in the world today. We shall examine some of their more picturesque manifestations in the pages that follow.

2

Fertility and Birth

IN his search for gods who could be held responsible for the success or failure of his enterprises, primitive Man endowed them with normal, human attributes. Perhaps the oldest myth of all was that concerned with the creation of man himself—that he had been conceived and born by the union of the great Sky Mother and Earth Father. During man's gradual transition from hunter to farmer, tilling the soil, growing crops and breeding stock for food and barter, the importance of fertility became paramount for survival. It is easy to see why the oldest customs and superstitions are concerned with fertility, but not necessarily man's own fertility or powers of pro-creation. The need for sexual activity, to conceive and produce children, was part of every-day life. But the success of the harvest and the fertility of livestock, depending largely on the elements, was a more doubtful matter. All possible precautions were taken against drought, poor crops and barrenness in breeding stock. The gods had to be propitiated. Sacrifices were made, and a whole ritual of behaviour carefully conducted to ensure success. The result was the gradual evolution of a whole series of fertility rites and customs concerned with the harvest, and found in all parts of the world. In the western hemisphere it was associated mainly with corn or barley, and in the Orient with rice. In almost every such superstition the spirit of fertility is thought to reside in the very last sheaf of the harvest, becoming the Corn Mother, Harvest Mother, or merely the Great Mother, according to the community. Crop fertility was closely linked with human fertility, and many harvest customs have an obvious reference to marriage and fertility in the community. But this was not the main aim of the fertility rites. They were essentially to please the gods and to ensure the continuance of plentiful crops. Their application to human fertility was only secondary.

The spirit of fertility, existing in the crop, was often represented in human form. In Brittany, for example, the last sheaf of corn was carefully shaped in the form of a woman, and a smaller, baby sheaf placed inside it. Here, and in many other places, it was commonly

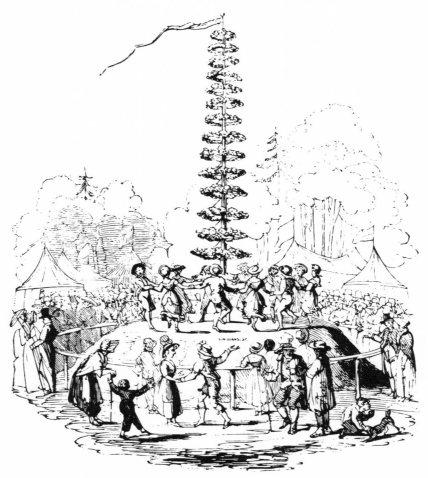

2 Maypole fertility dance

believed that whoever cut the last sheaf or was presented with the corn "dolly" would marry or produce a child before the next harvest. This could be a mixed blessing, and many a confirmed bachelor or mother of a large family took pains *not* to cut the last sheaf.

In Scotland and other parts of Europe the last sheaf was carefully preserved until the first mare had foaled, the god of fertility having expressed its approval by this sign. One of the strongest beliefs in the spirit of the harvest is found in Indonesia where it is believed that the rice crop actually has a soul. Also, the crop is treated exactly like a pregnant woman. It is watched over and prayed for, and no loud noises or disturbances are allowed which might interfere with the pregnancy. When the time comes for harvesting, the news is kept secret from the plant and a special language is used when discussing the harvest in the "hearing" of the rice. When harvesting begins a specially made small knife, which can be hidden in the hand, is used for the first cut so that the crop will suspect nothing, and the first two cuttings of the plant are fashioned into the shapes of a man and a woman. These are placed side-by-side in an ornate and decorated bed in a barn and must be left unseen and undisturbed for forty days.

If the encouragement of crop fertility could be achieved in this way, the demonstration of human sexual union might have even greater potency. Whether the gods of fertility lived in the sky, the mountains and trees, or in the crop itself, they had to be told what was wanted, and in no uncertain terms. So many primitive cults and religions included the sex act as part of the normal ritual. It was a holy and necessary thing and no stigma was attached to it. The profligacy and apparent debauchery that later took place at harvest and other festivals was not just a form of release of animal spirits; it had its roots in much deeper and more serious beliefs.

In many Eastern countries, and possibly among the Druids, sexual union was performed between priest and female acolyte, and later cultures extended it to the congregation. In some places it was confined to those who were married and had produced children, and those who had proved great fertility by producing triplets or twins. Among the Bugandas of Central Africa parents of twins are released from all normal village chores for a year. During this time they visit childless couples in the district, performing the sex act before them

23

in turn. Dances incorporating sexual union are also performed in the fields to encourage the plantain tree, the staple diet of the district, to flourish and bear fruit.

In pre-revolution Russia, at the spring sowing of the corn, those responsible habitually paired-off when the sowing was completed

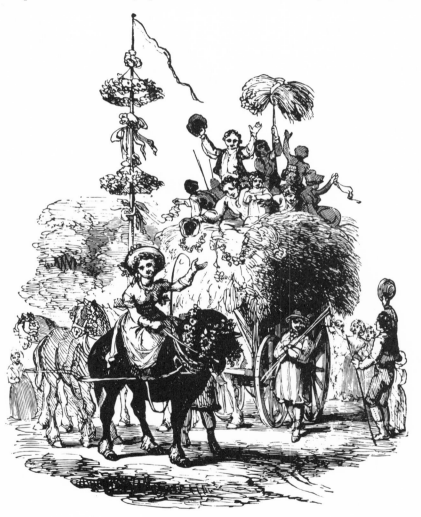

3 Bringing in the harvest

and rolled and tumbled in the newly-planted field while the priest blessed the proceedings. In the Ukraine the priest himself was expected to take part, and in Germany in the nineteenth century similar customs prevailed, but usually after harvest.

In Central South Africa it was a strict religious duty for couples to have intercourse just as the new seed was sown. In Java and Borneo the farmer and his wife had to visit each field in turn at night for the same purpose. Failure to do this would result in a poor crop, or even no crop at all, and was severely punished. Shortage of food would hurt the whole community. To help couples perform their sexual function adequately some communities imposed a rule of chastity during the actual period of sowing. Even today, some North American Indians sleep apart from their wives and eat no meat for fourteen days while seed is being sown. A similar custom prevails in several parts of Australia among the aborigines.

These fertility rites, harking back to the most ancient religious thought, have been held to survive in the sexual symbolism of much of the ritual of modern witchcraft, whose exponents see themselves as adherents of the "old religion" of pre-Christian times.

Efforts to ensure human fertility were understandably closely bound with the fertility of crops and animals. In many rural and agricultural communities to this day it is considered desirable that there should be a constant series of births in farm and family throughout the year. The idea was expressed in the remark of a Buckinghamshire farmer who maintained that "every female on the farm ought to be pregnant, including the missus." But this is an ideal that few find possible, or even desirable. Farmers' wives do not normally subscribe to this point of view.

The inability to produce a child has always been a matter of disgrace in less sophisticated communities, and every kind of "cure" has been used to help the barren woman. Superstitions to ensure the fertility of the new bride are found everywhere. Many still exist whose original purpose has long been forgotten. The throwing of rice at weddings, or the more modern version of confetti, is rooted in the belief that the fertility of the plant is grafted on to the person who comes in contact with it. The wedding cake itself is a symbol of fruitfulness. In some countries a piece of the cake is thrown out of the window the moment it is cut. If it shatters into fragments on impact it is a sign of many children, but if it remains in one piece the luckless bride will remain barren. For the same reason it is considered essential that the first slice should be cut by the bride and not by the groom. In the Middle East the orange has long been a symbol of fertility, and the traditional orange-blossom worn by western brides perpetuates this superstition.

But superstitions to ensure fertility are not only linked with plants. In many parts of eastern Europe a woman who fails to conceive within a reasonable time after marriage is beaten with a stick that has been used to separate copulating dogs. By this means the fertility of the animal is transferred to the human. More obscure is the theory that contact with the dead body of a criminal will induce fertility. In seventeenth-century England the hands or feet of a gallows corpse were often cut off and hurried to the home of a childless woman.

At an early stage it was realized that the inability to produce a child was not always the fault of the woman. She may have had several children by one man, and none by another. Frequently the fault in the man was thought to be an insufficiently large penis, and in Brazil it is customary for a man so afflicted to belabour his organ with the branches of the *aninga*, a prolific and luxuriant plant growing on the river bank. Many ancient writers, including the Chinese, believed that sexual excess was the cause of infertility, and medical writers through the ages constantly recommend a cessation of intercourse for a spell, after which conception is more likely to occur. The Russian version of this cure stresses the fact that during this interval the husband should not indulge in any extra-marital intercourse, as the process is designed to augment *his* virility. In Russia, as in many other countries, infertility and impotence were coupled with improper diet, and in particular with incomplete elimination of the bowels. Enemas and douches were used to cure the condition, and even today in the western world "colonic irrigation," by which the colon is flushed out with gallons of water under pressure, remains a popular treatment, particularly in America. Here, as in so many aspects of folk-medicine, we are on the narrow borderline dividing superstition and science, for more than one case has been recorded of an apparently infertile woman being able to conceive after this treatment.

Certain herbs are held to be specifics against infertility, and may have some scientific basis when taken internally. Harder to accept are the claims made for these same plants, among which the willow has pride of place, when merely placed beneath the conjugal bed. Similarly, the keeping of a small species of fig in pots around the house was also said to create a fertile atmosphere.

Many nostrums were available to childless couples, a typical sample was a "Mixture to Promote Breeding" printed in *The Compleat*

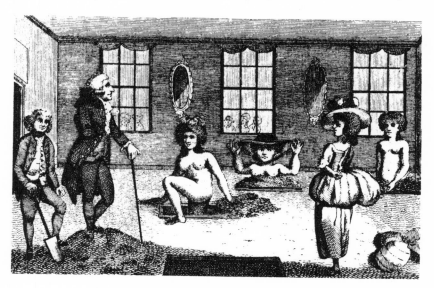

4 "Bathing in earth" (Dr. James Graham)

Housewife in London in 1753. This started from a basis of three pints of strong ale in which was boiled three "ox-backs" (presumably the spinal marrow of the animal), catmint and other garden herbs, sliced dates, stoned raisins, three whole nutmegs "prick'd full of holes" and the "syrup of stinking orris." This mixture had to be taken each night, but out of sight of the husband. There were strict instructions, while drinking, to "remain very cheerful and let nothing disquiet you." Eighteenth-century England was rife with herbalists and quack-merchants of every kind, and many so-called medical practitioners made fortunes out of herbs and charms to ward off infertility. One of the most famous was "Dr." James Graham, born in Edinburgh in 1745, and one of the first to cash in on early experiments with electricity and magnetism. During the 1780s he became famous throughout Europe for his sumptuous Temple of Health situated in Adelphi Terrace, just off the Strand in London. Here, in a spectacular setting, he demonstrated the advantages obtainable from Health, Sex and Beauty. He gave his celebrated lectures on the interrelation of the three subjects, attracting vast crowds (after payment of 2 gns entrance fee) and illustrating his lectures with the assistance of bevies of beautiful and scantily-clad girls he called his Goddesses of Health. A "recruitment advertisement" for this somewhat equivocal position ran as follows:

"WANTED. *Genteel, decent, modest young woman; she must be personally agreeable, blooming, healthy and sweet-tempered and well recommended for modesty, good sense and steadiness. She is to live in the Physician's family, to be daily dressed in white silk robes with a rich rose coloured girdle. If she can sing, play on the harpsichord or speak French greater wages will be given. Enquire Dr. Graham, Adelphi Temple.*"

The good doctor had little trouble in gaining recruits. One of them, a sixteen-year-old girl called Emma Lyons, later became famous as Lady Hamilton, the mistress of Admiral Lord Nelson. But the most spectacular and original contribution to health and well-being made by Graham at his Temple of Health was his extraordinary Grand Celestial Bed. This was guaranteed to ensure pregnancy for any woman who spent a night in it with her man, and though Graham himself advertised the nightly charge as £50 it is known that many noblemen paid as much as £500 to spend a blissful evening within its curtained and aromatic fastness. No feathers were used for the mattresses, but sweet new straw mingled with balm, rose leaves, flowers of lavender and oriental spices. In addition, and harking back to the principle of "imitative therapy," hair from the tails of full-blooded stallions was also used to ensure no lack of virility to the male member using it. But the chief attribute of the Celestial Bed (sometimes called The Electro-Magnetico Bed because of the 15 cwt of "compound magnets" built into it) was its ability to move on its axis or pivot and assume almost any angle. This was really quite exceptional and once again we find ourselves on the borderline between quackery and science, for it is just possible that the tilting of the bed at the required angle might induce sperm to reach the uterus where it had never penetrated before. But let the good doctor himself describe the advantages of his bed :

"Should pregnancy at any time not happily ensue I have the most astonishing method to recommend which will infallibly produce a genial and happy issue, I mean my Celestial or Magnetico-Electrico bed, which is the first and only ever in the world : it is placed in a spacious room to the right of my orchestra which produces the Celestial fire and the vivifying influence : this brilliant Celestial Bed is supported by six massive brass pillars with Saxon blue and purple satin, perfumed with Arabian spices in the style of those in the Seraglio of the Grand Turk. Any lady or gentleman desirous of progeny, and wishing to spend an evening in the Celestial apartment, after coition may, by a complement of a £50 bank note, be permitted to partake of the heavenly joys it affords by causing immediate conception, accompanied by soft music. Superior ecstasy which the parties enjoy in the Celestial Bed is really astonishing and never before thought in this world : the barren must certainly become fruitful when they are powerfully agitated in the delights of love."

The bed is said to have cost Graham £10,000, and it certainly seems to have been an astonishing contrivance, though unfortunately there is no record of its efficacy. Some even cast doubts on its value as a means of conception, and the writer Horace Walpole referred to it as "the most impudent puppet-show of imposition" he had ever seen. The Temple of Health attracted enormous crowds. Nevertheless Graham's overheads must have been heavy, for he later moved to a new Temple in a cheaper locality off Pall Mall, at that time bordering on the country. Here the "doctor" continued advertising the advantages of his famous bed and crowds flocked to hear his lectures in which he gave instructions for retaining virility and, in an age when personal hygiene was scarcely thought of, advocated thorough washing "from the top of the head to the end of the most distant toe" as a vital precursor to sexual intercouse. He was also very much against the use of double beds, describing them as a form of "matrimonial whoredom." He thundered against fornication and masturbation, and was before his time in demanding the removal of prostitutes from the streets. Even more remarkable, he advocated reducing taxes for those who produced several children and demanded compulsory sterilization of those who had inherited disease. But though many of these ideas were to be accepted later, the time was not yet ripe and the public tired of Graham. He made a final attempt at a come-back in premises in Panton Street, near London's Haymarket, where he preached the gospel of earth-bathing and allowed himself to be buried in soil up to the chin, bravely lecturing at the same time. But the public was bored, and Graham finally went back to Edinburgh where he died in 1794 having become a victim of a religious mania in his last years.

Graham made a fortune out of the contemporary preoccupation with sex, but he frowned on the use of aphrodisiacs as an artificial stimulant. Where failure to conceive is thought to be due to lack of sexual activity in the male (or, less common, in the woman) many things have been used to rectify this state of affairs and thought to have sexually-stimulating properties. Probably the most famous of these in the history of medicine is *cantharides*, a product made from the powdered bodies of a species of fly which infests certain trees in Spain and Portugal, and gives it its popular name of "Spanish Fly". Its action as an aphrodisiac derives from the irritation produced in the urogenital tract even in minute quantities. As irritation is produced in other parts of the body, notably the gullet and bowels, it is a highly dangerous substance and can easily prove fatal. In 1967 a London man inadvertently killed a girl at an office party when he put some cantharides into her drink, though it is not normally obtainable over the counter. Since about 1938 it has been rigidly controlled as a Dangerous Drug. Prior to that, however, it could be sold in pharmacies as long as it was intended for use only on animals, and was a favourite amongst rabbit-breeders despite the notorious aptitude of these animals for sexual activity in their normal state. It is also said to have a beneficial action in stimulating the growth of hair, and in a minute quantity in combination with bay rum is still used by those fearing premature baldness. Many other substances have been thought to stimulate sexual desire, including derivatives of marihuana, but most have been shown to be completely valueless. Certain foods are said to have sex-rousing properties, notably oysters, anchovies, steaks and spinach, but there is no scientific basis for this belief.

A plant long held to have magical and aphrodiasical powers is the mandrake, whose divided root bears some resemblance to a human form. It is said to stimulate sexual activity and promote fertility. The mandrake has the rare distinction of having its powers mentioned in the Bible (*Genesis*: 30, 14-17), when the childless Rachel begs Leah to give her some of the plant. Rachel's later delivery of a son, Joseph, is attributed to God rather than to the root, but the story does show the great antiquity of the mandrake legend. In France and Germany it was supposed to grow where a criminal had died and in some countries was said to glow at night. The most spectacular attribute of the plant, however, was its capacity to utter a piercing shriek when it was removed from the ground. Better authenticated was its use in syrup as a cure for insomnia and as a general anaesthetic, and at least one modern manufacturer uses the active ingredient of mandrake as the basis of sleeping-tablets.

Drugs which genuinely stimulate sexual activity are virtually unknown and the effect of those said to do so remains largely in the mind. The effect of alcohol in this respect is a typical example. Because of its deadening effect on the control area of the brain, alcohol is often regarded as a stimulant. In fact it is a sedative, and though it may stimulate the imagination and the desire for sex it reduces sexual performance, as prostitutes well know. Prostitution itself has played its part in the age-long search for fertility. In certain communities in pre-Christian times it was considered essential that every young girl should sell herself for a short period before marriage to ensure fertility. This was not looked on as sinful or lustful. On the contrary, it was a solemn religious rite practised, as in Cyprus, before the temple of Aphrodite. In Babylon every woman, whatever her status, had to offer herself at least once for money to a stranger, and dedicate the proceeds to the priests of the temple. Only in this way could she be sure of a full and happy family life.

The union of man and woman in marriage is seen in most communities not just as a physical union, but a mental one too. The many beliefs and superstitions surrounding the pregnant wife, particularly during her confinement, often involve the husband. Few of these beliefs are more long-standing than the idea that the husband must suffer, as his wife suffers, during the period of pregnancy. This theory, found the world over, is often referred to as the *couvade*, and persists even today. Modern husbands, whose wives are pregnant, have only to mention a minor discomfort, such as backache, for it to be attributed to their wife's condition and to find themselves the butt of jokes and leg-pulling on the part of friends and acquaintances. But in many primitive societies the matter was taken very seriously. During the wife's pregnancy it was often the man who retired to bed, and it was to the husband and not the wife that gifts were brought. The husband's "illness" during this period was thought to be in direct proportion to the affection in which he held his wife, and his complete prostration was held to be evidence of a true undying love. The *couvade* could also be used to determine the paternity of an illegitimate child, and as recently as the nineteenth century, in England, when an unmarried girl gave birth to a child the locals would at once search the village for a man who was ill, naming him as the father. Recovery, in many cases, was immediate!

Many were the customs and superstitions devoted to easing delivery and reducing the labour of the expectant mother. Once again we meet imitative therapy. To allow unimpeded and easy delivery of the child there must be nothing near at hand which could be considered blocked-up or restrained in any way. All doors and windows were opened at the moment of birth, and any knots were untied. In some societies this superstition extends to the whole period of pregnancy, and the woman is forbidden to tie up anything or to make a knot in case it prevents the eventual free delivery of the child. In its most extreme form the midwife, just before attending the confinement, opens every door in the house, uncorks every bottle or jar and even unties every cow, sheep or horse on the premises. In many areas it is forbidden to sit cross-legged in the presence of a pregnant woman, for this will assuredly cause trouble for her later. In eighteenth-century Scotland it was the custom to loosen every fastening in the clothes of bride and groom before the wedding ceremony so that there should be no bar to procreation. Conversely the superstition could be invoked in a malevolent manner, and it was well known that to make a bridegroom impotent one only had to tie a knot in a handkerchief and hide it in one of his pockets. In some areas the knotted handkerchief had to be thrown into water, but in either case the husband would be unable to father a child until the knot became undone.

Assuming that the happy couple survived such antisocial behaviour, and the wife reached the end of her term some nine months later, the actual birth too was attended by much folklore and superstition. The day of the week was a sign of the future fate of the infant, a belief still alive and perpetuated in the old rhyme beginning.

> *Monday's child is fair of face,*
> *Tuesday's child is full of grace.*

The hour, too, was of vital importance, and still remains a most relevant item in the divination of the future by means of astrology. Babies born at midnight have the gift of second-sight and those born at dusk are said to be able to see ghosts. Birth by Caesarian section has long been held to forecast strength and bounding health in later life, and in some parts of the world a child who is born feet foremost is destined to be a mighty traveller and thought to have magical powers. The presence of the caul at birth is considered a specific against death by drowning and it is said that even today sailors will pay large amounts to obtain cauls to keep with them.

But not all the accidents of birth are of necessity beneficial to the infant. In parts of Africa it is believed that if a child is born on the first day of the second month of the year, its house will be burned down. To avoid this, the neighbours build a rough shed nearby and set it on fire, to circumvent the catastrophe. For it to be really effective the mother and newborn child should first be placed inside the substitute "home" and rescued only when the flames have gained a hold.

Circumstances of birth can also endow the infant with special gifts, particularly those of healing. A posthumous child was popularly supposed to have the power of curing thrush by breathing on the victim, and the seventh child of a seventh child was considered to have the power of healing a great variety of diseases. In cases of scrofula, or King's Evil, the touch by such a person was considered as valuable as the royal touch itself, and it was just as effective in healing goitre.

In many parts of Europe a newborn child is quickly carried upstairs in order that he may rise in life and gain advancement. Sometimes he is given his first bath before a fire of ashwood, as legend says that the infant Jesus was first bathed before such a fire. Presumably also connected with early Christian belief is the custom of ensuring that the first person to nurse the child should be a virgin, a practice still sometimes found in the north of England.

But what of the mother? She has carried out her function and ceases to be the focus of attention. In some communities she is regarded as unclean, and in Tahiti has to spend the next three weeks alone in a hut away from the village, out of contact with other women, until pure again. In South Africa both child and mother are considered unclean for a long period, and the father is thought to be at risk if he handles his child within three months of birth. In Alaska a woman who is about to give birth is also set apart and fed with sticks so that no-one may be contaminated by her.

In civilized societies, traces of these ancient beliefs still remain. Many women continue to oppose the easing of the natural process of childbirth, believing it to be both sinful and medically unjustified. In country areas, even today, a woman having her monthly period may be warned not to cut meat until the flow is over—a lingering relic of the belief that she is unclean during this time. The personal problems of menstruation, pregnancy and birth are still regarded by many women as unsuitable for open discussion, and while this attitude lingers superstition and old wives' tales will continue to exert their influence and create confusion.

3

Contraception and Abortion

ALL cultures aimed at the ideal of maximum fertility in crops and farm animals. But the same objective was not always desired for the human members of the community. From the earliest times family planning has been practised, though the reasons for this differed according to the culture and social habits of the community.

In her fascinating book *The Jungle Search for Nature's Cures* the American writer Nicole Maxwell tells how, in the jungles of Peru, a root is gathered and a decoction made from it to avoid pregnancy after intercourse. One cupful of the mixture will make a woman infertile, and recourse to this is often had by Indian women whose husbands are unsympathetic to them, or have unpleasant characteristics, in order that these attributes are not perpetuated in any children of the marriage. Should the wife leave her husband, marry again and desire children, another root is used, again in only a single dose. This would make the wife fertile once more. A third root is used to procure an abortion if required, though its power is less remarkable than that of the other two plants, which are hard to identify, and are jealously guarded by the tribes concerned. Even when these roots were at last identified it was pointed out that they would be unlikely to work without the magic incantations or songs. The balance between population and food supplies is often the reason for limiting family size. The unforeseen failure of a crop may precipitate untold hardship in one year, but normally the balance is held so that over a period there is enough food for all. This is achieved partly by direct human agency and partly by the self-regulating effect of the environment. Where malnutrition exists and disease is rife the effect is to induce infertility often in both men and women. In some areas of Africa more than half the female population may be barren, largely owing to tuberculosis and gonorrhoea. Even where so much infertility does not exist, and where conditions are good, the number of children produced by primitive peoples is surprisingly small. Taking the potential child-bearing life of a woman as the thirty years between fifteen and forty-five, one might assume that a total of ten or twelve children during this period is not excessive. Yet no primitive peoples even approach this figure. Among the Sioux Indians the average number of children is eight, while amongst the Eskimos, where conditions are certainly arduous, the average drops to five. Even accounting for miscarriages and a fairly high mortality rate it seems that in many cases the women of primitive tribes are in a state of pregnancy far less often than are many of their civilized sisters. But there are other factors which produce this result. One is the widespread custom of suckling infants for two or even three years. During this period sexual intercourse may be forbidden by man-made taboos. But where lactation is heavy and prolonged, ovulation may be decreased, and with it the chance of conceiving again quickly. We should remember, too, that primitive peoples are far less sexually inclined than are their civilized counterparts. Animals, in their wild state, are far less sexually active than in captivity and a study of the mating habits of the gorilla in the wild indicates that the male may go for several months without having intercourse. The famous Kinsey report of 1953 showed that among white American women in the age-groups 16 to 20 intercouse took place an average of 3.7 times each week, dropping to 1.7 times in the 41 to 46 age group. This is far higher than in most primitive tribes, and it has also been noted that even civilized Negroes take three times as long as white people to reach orgasm. But in ancient civilized cultures —Egypt, Greece, Rome—intercourse took place more often and artificial means had to be adopted to avoid procreation. More than three thousand years ago the Ebers papyrus describes a contraceptive pessary containing a sperm-killing agent, in this case asses' milk. But not until the end of the nineteenth century was the value of lactic acid as a spermicide finally proved. Other methods were also in vogue in ancient Egypt including the smearing of a resinous gum over the mouth of the womb to form a purely physical barrier. Nearer to the contraceptive pastes popular in our own day was the mixture of honey and soda inserted in the vagina, while yet another method was associated with what has been termed "sewerage pharmacology"—the use of crocodile and other dung to make a contraceptive pessary. An interesting method of contraception described in a papyrus of 1550 B.C. consists of soaking a piece of cloth in honey in which the powdered leaves of the acacia tree have been mixed. This is then used as a tampon. Once again we find the system based on scientific fact, for fermenting acacia leaves produce lactic acid.

The Egyptian preoccupation with contraception was not based on economies or a shortage of food supplies. In a culture devoted to the admiration of the beautiful it was more likely to have been caused by a desire to preserve the beauty of the female figure and to allow women to look young as long as possible. In Roman times the problem was dealt with in far less sophisticated ways. Indeed, the literature of the age is remarkable in having few references to chemical or physical methods of contraception. In a society noted for its sexual licence, where both men and women were notoriously unfaithful and where it was not unusual for the Roman matron to copulate with her slave, two basic methods were used to avoid the responsibility of children. Either the slave was made sterile by surgery, or the infant was killed at birth. The Roman midwife was a woman of many parts. Not only was she expected to reduce the birth-pangs of her mistress when her time came, but also to be expert in the removal of the newly-born and its instant disposal. She was an accomplished poisoner and an expert in the concoction of aphrodisiacs. Her main value was often as an abortionist, and so successful were these women that by 164 B.C. the population of Rome was found to be declining at an alarming rate. Indeed, the Censor, Quintus Metellus, was forced to urge new laws to keep up the birth-rate. These included inducements to couples to have large families and penalties for those who remained celibate. They did little good, and the downfall of the Roman empire has been attributed by some writers to the results of sexual promiscuity coupled with the apparently paradoxical fall in the population.

The Greek attitude to sex and contraception was far more sophisticated. Both in Sparta and in Athens marital union was designed as a source of virile male children who could one day fight in the Greek armies. Weak and sickly children, particularly females, were left to die. Infanticide was very common. The Greeks were well aware of the danger of over-population, however, and Plato was probably the first writer to give serious thought to legal methods of limiting the size of families. He suggested in his *Republic* that men should be allowed to father children only between the ages of 25 and 35 and women to conceive only between 20 and 40. In his ideal state the population would be carefully held in check and not allowed to exceed 5,040. Abortion and infanticide would be legalized, and citizens would surrender all their rights for the common good of the community.

In Plato's Greece the very way of life militated against a high birth-rate, for homosexuality was normal and the adolescent Greek youth became the lover of an older man as a matter of course, marrying a woman only later in life and producing the required number of children. The ideal of "Platonic friendship" was thus originally a homosexual one, and Plato's young pupils, grouped around their master's knee during the day, took it as a matter of course that tuition did not cease at nightfall. Women in Greek society were not to be envied. They were treated merely as vehicles for growing the seed implanted in them by their lord if they were married, or, if unmarried, as a means of gratifying sexual desire. There were three grades of prostitute, the highest being the "intimate female companion," beautiful, clever, proficient in the arts of music and dancing, and achieving the highest prestige amongst Greek women. With women of this kind pregnancy could be a social calamity, and it is not surprising that many methods of contraception are described in Greek literature.

Aristotle, with his wife Pythias, in particular seems to have studied various types of contraceptive techniques including the use of oil to cover the vagina. He also advocated the ingestion of the bodies of certain spiders for this purpose. Hippocrates, or more accurately writers of the Hippocratic school (for there are virtually no surviving authentic writings of Hippocrates himself) first mentioned an appliance which bears some resemblance to the modern intra-uterine device. This was a hollow lead tube filled with mutton-fat; it was inserted into the womb, presumably with the object of keeping it open. Today we know that any foreign object, of almost any shape, introduced into the uterus will inhibit conception, but the exact reason for this is still not clear.

The Hippocratic writers also mentioned various contraceptive drinks, one of which was supposed to prevent conception for a year. Unfortunately the substances used in this potion cannot be identified. One of them, called Cyprian, is equated with Chalcitis from Egypt, but apart from the comment that the latter is "good for fluxes of blood coming from the womb" there is no further clue as to what this substance was.

Other and later writers, such as Dioscorides, who lived in the second century A.D., are more specific. Mention is made of various substances which could be used as spermicides. They include, once again, lactic acid—this time in the form of pomegranate juice. They also recommended that after intercouse a woman should at once rise, sneeze, wipe out her vagina, and drink something cold. Great importance was attached to making violent bodily contortions after intercourse, to try and dislodge the male sperm. Mention is made of the contraceptive properties of white lead, a substance eaten in large quantities by the priestesses of the temples in ancient China, where sexual intercourse was part of the religious ceremony, and who also burned herbs on their bellies for the same purpose.

Men used many methods to avoid fertilization, for example washing the penis in vinegar or brine before insertion. This had some scientific basis. Less appropriate were methods involving association with infertile animals, such as mules; the old prescription of drinking a mixture containing the pulverized testicles of that animal to induce male sterility could not have been very effective. Less effective still were the charms and amulets recommended even by those compara-tively erudite writers whose studies were leading them somewhere towards the truth.

The best way of reducing the chances of pregnancy is, and always has been the simple device of abstention. Understandably unpopular it could only be imposed by means of laws, such as the Mosaic Laws relating to menstruation, during which intercourse was forbidden. The medical idea behind this was that fertility was greatest during this time and conception most likely—a theory now known to be false.

39

Midway between the use of contraceptives with complete sexual union, and total abstention, was a method used by almost all cultures—*coitus interruptus*. The Jewish Law regarding the continuance of the family even after the death of the father, by a brother of the dead man impregnating the widow, was, in fact, the legalizing of a custom found all over the world. The sin of Onan, who was called upon to perform this duty with Tamar, his dead brother's widow, and who purposely spilled his seed on the ground (*Genesis* 38, 7-10) is held by some scholars to refer to *coitus interruptus*. But this was "evil in the sight of the Lord, and the Lord slew him"—an argument used to prove the sinfulness of this form of contraception and of masturbation. The early Christian Church used this much-misunderstood text to show the sin of trying to avoid the normal results of intercourse, showing a confusion of thought that was to have far-reaching effects and create untold misery and squalor for many centuries to come. In the light of modern knowledge it seems far more likely that Onan's real sin was trying to avoid fertilizing Tamar, so that he would not have the legal responsibility for a child. This would be a crime against the Jewish Law of the time, though one may only hazard a guess at the true reasons that motivated Onan.

After the medical writings of the second century A.D. there is little recorded information on contraception and pregnancy for the next seven hundred years. It was the invasion of Europe by the Moslems that eventually allowed new learning and medical thought to permeate westwards, mainly through the writings of Rhazes and Avicenna, both working in Persia in the tenth century. Theirs is a much more enlightened attitude, particularly in regard to contraception, which is strongly advocated if pregnancy might place the women's life at risk. Many ancient techniques are described to avoid conception, and Rhazes recommends the use of convulsive and sudden movements to dislodge the foetus. He advises either seven or nine backward jumps to bring this about, a typical example of the mystique of medicine, for both seven and nine were numbers with "magic" qualities.

Astringent pessaries for use after intercourse are also described. Most of them contain sal ammoniac and potash. There are also such doubtful rituals as sitting on one's toes and stroking the navel with the thumb. An ancient Greek belief is repeated—that the womb is itself a separate and living being within the body that could move about at will. It was thought to be attracted by pleasant perfumes and odours and repelled by offensive smells. Fumigation of the vagina by evil-smelling herbs was therefore standard practice to cause the womb to move away from the site of the sperm, while the inhalation and smelling of perfumed vapours had a similar effect from above. The theory of "wandering womb" persisted well into the Middle Ages and a relic of it still exists in the word "hysteria" to denote a neurotic condition. It was thought that if the womb (the *hysterium*) wandered too far up in the body it would eventually affect the brain, and induce disorder.

Many of these contraceptive techniques proved of little value, and the next step was to induce abortion. Rhazes suggests various physical methods including the insertion into the vagina of a tube of paper or soft wood. This method remained a favourite, though highly danger-ous, device until the twentieth century, and up to World War Two and even later chemists were often asked to supply long strips of quassia bark for this purpose. Knitting needles were also extensively used by amateur abortionists, though the risks of perforation of the uterus and resultant septicaemia were great. The value of violent movement to effect abortion has long been favoured, and Rhazes himself advises this and in addition recommends "laughing and joking" to induce it. The humour of the situation is usually lost on the pregnant woman. But even today, in some country areas and in the crowded slums of big cities, jumping or sliding downstairs at midnight, preferably after drinking several gins, is superstitiously considered a specific. (In fact the physical shock, together with the presence of alcohol, may well bring about an abortion.)

Methods of inducing abortion by medicinal and herbal compounds abound in the writings of these tenth-century physicians. Most are valueless, though at a later age ergot became popular since it could act on the sphincter muscle of the uterus, and force it open. Its success was limited, for should the muscle already be open the drug can close it, a fact still occasionally used in modern gynaecology and obstetrics.

For those who disliked these drastic and doubtful methods of contraception, but wished merely to abstain from intercourse, lettuce was a favourite anaphrodisiac used to lessen sexual desire. The old idea that the menstrual flow indicates the presence of female eggs waiting to be fertilized was repeated, and it was advised not to have intercourse near this time. It was also recommended that partners in the sexual act should try and avoid the climacteric at the same time.

The writings of Rhazes and Avicenna remained the main source of medical information for the next five hundred years. Yet the information supplied would have been known only to those educated enough to read. Among the common people the old beliefs and superstitions persisted. Not that such beliefs were essentially different from the findings of the scholars, for such men had to a large extent merely crytallized and rendered into permanent form medical folklore that had existed for centuries. The medieval midwife, though less concerned with abortion, was a worthy successor to her Greek and Roman counterparts and had accumulated a wealth of knowledge which she guarded jealously. Indeed, that great fifteenth-century physician Paracelsus, who so disdained traditional methods of medicine that he publicly burned the works of Avicenna, had to admit that he had learned more of pregnancy and child-birth from the local midwives than he had ever done from the ancient writers. Paracelsus, and his near-contemporary the Flemish surgeon Vesalius, like all innovators, had a hard time gaining acceptance for their theories. During the sixteenth and seventeenth centuries knowledge of contraception seems almost to have taken a backward step. We hardly find any mention of vaginal douches or contraceptive pessaries. Reliance was placed mainly on decoctions of herbs taken orally and even those researchers who rediscovered the value of vinegar as a spermicide were ignored. Despite advances in anatomy and a truer understanding of the function of the female genitalia, little progress was made. One man who made a particular study of the female reproductive organs was the sixteenth-century anatomist Gabriel Fallopius, from whose name the fallopian tubes are derived. But Fallopius was also concerned with disease, especially with diseases of a sexual origin such as syphilis, and evolved a simple linen condom to be worn over the penis as a safeguard against infection. It was found to be quite effective, especially when later physicians advocated soaking the sheath in chemicals before use. Soon it was found that use of the condom (a word first used in England) also reduced the risk of pregnancy, and from that moment its popularity was assured. Like most great inventions it cannot be attributed to one man and a vast amount of folklore and legend has attended its origins. The sheath as a form of contraceptive was certainly in use in Paris in 1655, but not everyone was equally enthusiastic about it. Madame de Sévigné described it as "an armour against enjoyment and a spider's web against danger."

In England, too, condoms were felt to be a mixed blessing. But when the linen condom gave way to the sheath manufactured from the blind gut of a sheep, treated with chemicals and softened and dried, a booming trade began in London and spread to Paris, Berlin and even St. Petersburg. In London the centre of the trade was around Leicester Square, where the notorious and outrageous Mrs. Philips made a fortune in her premises in the eighteenth century and bombarded the public with advertising leaflets. She soon had competition, and at one period three "genuine" Mrs. Philipses were all indulging in cut-throat competition in the same street for the sale of condoms.

It is from this period that the most persistent story emerges as to their origin. It is said that an Irish chemist in London, a Joseph Condon, invented the sheath for the sole purpose of avoiding infection. When he found his invention was used mainly as a contraceptive his shame was such that he was forced to sell his business, change his name, and retire, broken and disillusioned, to his native Dublin. No justification for this tale has ever emerged, nor is it likely to do so as the use of condoms as contraceptives was first noted at least a century before. But the device, now in its more sophisticated latex form a fraction of a millimetre thick, still sells by the million in pharmacies, drug-stores and hairdressers. Their arrival precipitated criticism both from the Church and from those concerned with problems of depopulation. Others criticized the condom for different reasons, one writer complaining that "the least hole will permit contagion, and again, it may happen that during coitus the membrane may tear by a strong strain."

It is interesting that, unlike most inventions claimed by several countries, the contraceptive sheath was always described in terms denoting a foreign origin in whatever country it was used. In England it became known as the French letter while in France it was called the English cap. The notorious Casanova referred to it as the English overcoat, and an illustration in an early edition of his *Memoirs* shows him testing one for holes by blowing it up before a delighted audience. The very short condom which covered only the end of the penis was known as the American tip.

In Britain, after the First World War, rubber goods were on sale on request in most pharmacies with the exception of the 1,200 branches of Boots, the retail chemists. This company, which apparently banned their sale on religious grounds, continued to display a curious facet of Victorian mentality in allowing the sale of Rendells and other pessaries for women while refusing to stock contraceptives for men. Not until 1965 was this policy ended, and even then it was a year or two before rubber goods were available at every branch.

Between 1919 and 1939 various brands of French letters were openly displayed in most pharmacies as well as in drug stores and hairdressers. They normally came packaged in threes, selling at 6d, 10d, or 2s 6d according to quality and thinness of latex used. Most expensive of all was the single-packaged washable condom which could be used several times. Because of its comparative thickness this type of sheath was not very popular, though for the timid it was useful in that the embarassment of purchase was made less frequent. Even today men are oddly reticent in asking for rubber goods from a female assistant. The sight of a man peering hesitantly through the windows of a pharmacy is usually a signal for the girl assistant to vanish while the manager steps forward and ostentatiously busies himself about the shop. Only then will the prospective purchaser enter and whisper his request. This no doubt explains the huge sales of French letters in the all-male ambience of the barber's shop.

From time to time efforts have been made to design a condom which gives added sensation despite the inevitable lack of physical contact. At the turn of the century the "tickler" condom was in vogue which included a hard appendage at the tip designed to give increased satisfaction to the female. The idea was not new, for in many African tribes it has long been the custom for the male to make a small slit in the skin of the penis and insert grains of gravel or sand which remain in place as the skin grows over. Similarly the custom of inserting a feather into the end of the penis for the same purpose is fairly common.

Despite insistence that condoms were of foreign origin, Victorian pride in Britain and the Empire was not to be slighted. In the 1880s rubber goods appeared on the market carrying highly-coloured portraits of the Liberal Prime Minister W. E. Gladstone, and Queen Victoria. There were many who felt this was stretching patriotism too far!

Not until the end of the nineteenth century did the chemical contraceptive pessary (mentioned by Aristotle) first come into vogue. In the meantime Victorian patent-medicine manufacturers did a roaring trade with a variety of nostrums including "sterility powder" for men and "female pills" for women, the latter designed to promote menstrual flow after intercourse. The Dutch cap, this time genuinely named as it was invented in Holland, engaged the attention of earnest gynaecologists, though the subject of contraception as a whole was discouraged in the medical press.

In 1880 W. J. Rendell, a chemist in Clerkenwell, London, produced the first commercial spermicidal pessary. It was a mixture of quinine and coco-butter made to melt at just above body-temperature and was an instant success. For the next ninety years these continued to be the stand-by of married women the world over and are still used as an alternative to the Pill. But the Pill itself, originating in the mysterious plants used by Mexican Indians, has almost replaced it, as have the various intra-uterine devices now available. The modern Pill is a highly-sophisticated hormonal product, but i.u.d.s are an ancient device which, despite much research, still refuse to reveal exactly how they work.

In its early days the Rendell pessary was bought by social workers and distributed free to the poor. A curious item of medical folklore was the rumour that, to comply with government regulations aimed at avoiding depopulation, one pessary in every box had to be a blank. There is some evidence that this notion was purposely put about by the anti-contraceptionists, in the hope that women would lose confidence and stop using them. If this was so the scheme backfired disastrously. Once the rumour spread the immediate result was that women began inserting two pessaries instead of one, to make quite sure they were protected, and sales virtually doubled! In the trade it was openly said that the whole idea was started by Rendells themselves, and was a stroke of genius on the part of their sales manager.

Information on contraception had spread in Europe and America during most of the nineteenth century despite active opposition from almost every religious body and government. In America, one of the early pioneers was Charles Knowlton, a New England doctor, whose book *The Fruits of Philosophy, or the Private Companion of Young Married People* was published anonymously in 1832. Knowlton began by demolishing the familiar argument that contraception was unnatural. He pointed out that the whole of civilization was a never-ending battle with the effects of uncontrolled natural processes. He stressed the advantages of limiting families, especially in poor environments, and pointed to the terrible health problems of women whose constitutions were weakened by constant pregnancies, miscarriages or abortions. Various means of circumventing conception were described, mainly with the use of chemical solutions by douching or by syringe. Such information was long overdue. Though many women were afraid to use any form of contraception that would have been apparent to their husbands, various forms of physical manipulation were indulged in afterwards to avoid pregnancy, and several "do-it-yourself" techniques were popular. Some included the use of potentially dangerous chemicals, such as the swallowing of pills made of plaster-of-lead, or drinking water in which copper coins had been boiled. Knowlton advocated the use of alum in solution or vinegar as a form of douche, both of which had been known to the ancients but forgotten for a thousand years.

Strangely enough, despite the importance of its controversial theme, *The Fruits of Philosophy* caused little comment in medical circles. Not until eleven years after publication was it reviewed by the *Boston Medical Journal*, which primly accused the author of advocating unnatural practices and said that the less the public knew about such things the better!

As so often happens it was litigation which created wide public interest in the subject. Knowlton was fined several times and eventually imprisoned for publishing "filth." Sales soared. His book was published in England the same year it appeared in America, but once again it was barely noticed and for the next forty years enjoyed a sale of only about seven hundred copies annually. Not until a new edition was published by the famous free-thinkers, Charles Bradlaugh and Annie Besant, in 1877, did the authorities act. There followed a testcase in the publication of contraceptive literature. So much publicity surrounded the arrest of the two defendants that between then and their trial three months later the book sold 125,000 copies. The authors were found guilty and sentenced to six months' imprisonment, but on appeal the conviction was quashed due to a technical error in the original indictment. The *Fruits of Philosophy* had achieved its purpose, though by the 1880s had become largely out-of-date. Even so it was still frowned upon by the authorities, and booksellers up and down the country were still being fined or even imprisoned for stocking it as late as 1892. By then its total sales had reached 300,000.

In America, where *The Fruits of Philosophy* had first seen the light, action against "indecent" literature was even more venomous. This was mainly due to the activities of Anthony Comstock, a Civil War veteran and Congressman, who in 1873 succeeded in introducing Section 221 of the Federal Code which provided heavy fines and imprisonment for anyone advertising contraceptive methods or sending such literature through the mails. For nearly half a century Comstock and his employees toured the countryside, swooping on booksellers, examining the mails and conducting a campaign against this "pornography" which was little short of obsessional. Typical of Comstock's technique was to enter a brothel as a prospective customer, ask to have various girls paraded nude in front of him, and then arrest them for indecent exposure. He died in 1915, lamented by few.

Despite Comstock and his minions American workers continued to spread the gospel of contraception and family planning. They included such stalwarts as Edward Bliss Foote, Burt Green Wilder and later Margaret Sanger and Emma Goldman. In Britain by far the most famous and controversial figure was to be Marie Stopes during the early years of the twentieth century. This difficult and obstinate woman opened Britain's first birth control clinic in London in 1921, backed by such famous figures as H. G. Wells, Arnold Bennett and Dame Clara Butt. Its work was hotly opposed, mainly by the Roman

Catholic Church, and in 1923 a libel action which she brought against Halliday Sutherland, a Catholic doctor who had criticized her work, became a cause célèbre. Though a jury found in her favour, Sutherland's appeal to the House of Lords was upheld, though, once again, publicity surrounding the litigation brought her more fame and supporters than she could have achieved on her own. The work of Marie Stopes led to the foundation of the National Birth Control Council in England in 1930, an organization better-known today as the Family Planning Association.

In these so-called permissive times the subjects of contraception and abortion are discussed openly, though they are still capable of arousing heated and emotional discussions. The provision of contraceptive devices under the National Health Service is now hotly debated and some of the arguments used against it are little different from those expressed a century ago. Comstockery, it seems, is not yet dead.

4

The Folklore of Infancy

WHETHER a child is born in the frozen wastes of Siberia, an African kraal, or in the civilized West, it is reasonable to suppose that both parents and relations are concerned in its welfare. During her pregnancy the mother will have taken such precautions as are felt necessary in her community. In this she will have had the benefit of much advice, for few events in her life will attract more interest in those around her, particularly from those who are themselves mothers.

In northern Europe, notably in Wales and Brittany, she may have been warned not to sew or knit during pregnancy, in case her child should one day be hanged. She will certainly have been advised not to exert herself too much during this period, and to follow a strict regimen of diet and hygiene. The effects of experiences and ideas sustained during pregnancy have long been associated with the well-being of the child. Ancient Chinese medical literature, for example, explains many illnesses of childhood in this way. The famous *Yellow Emperor's Classic of Internal Medicine*, embodying medical beliefs at least three thousand years old, states that the health of an infant is directly related to the successful combination of the sperm (*Ching*) and energy (*Ch'i*) in the mother's womb. Should this combination be disturbed by a sudden or unpleasant experience or shock the result may well be epilepsy in the infant. Beliefs far less less plausible than this abound to explain almost every infant ailment. Failure to adopt Dr. Emma Drake's precept to "look only at beautiful things" may well have tragic consequences. Looking at a wild hare may result in the child having a hare-lip, and watching the feeding habits of pigs may risk the child having a face like a pig, or at least sounding like one! Superstitions such as these are common, and die hard.

For those living by the sea the time of birth could be forecast with some exactitude, for it was related to the ebb and flow of the tide. Children, it was well known, were born only on the incoming tide, just as death took place only on the ebb. But even if the infant was born whole and healthy the risks in the first few months of its life were even greater than those in the womb. Above all, the child had to be protected from witches, for the witches' ability to fly depended on a plentiful supply of baby-fat with which to smear herself. But witches were afraid of iron, and in many European countries it was customary to drive large nails into the cradle to avoid this risk. Cats have long been thought harmful to babies and were popularly supposed to jump on the cot and "draw the breath" of the sleeping child until it expired. The mere presence of a cat around the house was often held responsible for illness in a child, and more than one unlucky cat has been done to death in an effort to effect a cure.

Despite instructions to the pregnant mother to keep her mind off unpleasant things, the very books meant to help her through this difficult period were often alarming in the extreme. *The Household Physician* of 1899 lists under "Common Diseases of Infancy" such terrifying afflictions as scrofula, consumption, water on the brain, paralysis and syphilis! The prognosis for a child that did not reach full term was poor indeed, and the "vulgar notion" that a child born at seven months was likely to be healthier than one born at eight months was severely scotched.

Most dangerous for a baby was the period between birth and baptism. It was then particularly vulnerable to the actions of spirits, both evil and good. While witches waited to snatch the child and boil it down for fat, fairies might also be about, only too eager to take the child and make it their own, substituting a changeling in its place.

As Christina Hole has pointed out in her *English Folklore* baptism illustrates a curious mixture of pagan and Christian beliefs. Both the Druids and the Norsemen held naming ceremonies, which not only protected the child from disease but also legalized its existence and gave it the right of inheritance. Even today, in some areas, when an unbaptized child is taken ill the mother will send to the church for a supply of "christening water" in an attempt to cure it Even if the newborn infant did not succumb from scrofula, water-on-the-brain or syphilis, it would almost certainly have to run the gauntlet of childhood diseases like measles, mumps and whooping-cough. Fortunately the child was not usually aware of the content of some of these prescriptions as, for example, the cure for whooping cough given in *The Compleat Housewife*: "Take a spoonful of wood-lice, bruise them, mix them with breast milk and taken three or four mornings as you find benefit. It will cure, but some must take longer than others."

Cures for whooping-cough ("chin-cough" in some districts) are many and various. "Swing the child upwards by the heels" was one valuable precept, though a commoner if less strenuous prescription was to pass the child under and over a donkey. Obtaining a ferret, giving it milk to drink, and feeding the unconsumed portion to the child, was another remedy, while other folk pinned their faith on administering onion-juice to the soles of the feet. A curious custom still found in urban areas is to carry the patient around the gasworks! In 1950 the *Guardian* reported a serious outbreak of whooping-cough in Hertfordshire with anxious parents solemnly marching round the local Eastern Gas Board plant with infants at the ready. The newspaper attributed this procedure to a rather too literal interpretation of the doctors' recommendation for a "change of air," though the reason may well have been connected with the presence of coal-tar derivatives thought to be present in the atmosphere. A similar reasoning is found in the custom of taking a victim of whooping-cough to a place where the road is being tarred. Whether or not such cures were effective (and there are many mothers who insist they were) they make better sense than the use of "transference" rituals such as putting a fish in the child's mouth and then throwing the fish into the river to transfer the illness to the other fish. Death from whooping-cough is virtually unknown today. But this is quite a recent thing, and as late as 1895 a medical guide-book, after giving instructions for treatment, concluded with the cheering remark that "though recovery *ought* to take place, death may occur during a spasm."

Based on sound scientific principles are the many cures for ringworm involving metal. The favourite was to obtain an axe-head, heat it over a flame until it began to "sweat" and then collect the exudation and immediately apply it to the affected part. In modern medicine one of the most effective treatments for this disease makes use of metallic salts, mainly those of copper.

To ward off coughs and colds small bags of camphor were hung around the necks of toddlers, though to cure a cough garlic was a favourite remedy. Garlic was also used in the treatment of worms, another curse of infancy. Though aloes was taken internally (and still is) this vegetable was often used more as a diagnostic than a therapeutic substance. To find out if worms were still present an eighteenth-century medical book gives instructions for making a paste of powdered aloes and lard. This was spread on a piece of flannel and applied to the child's navel. If it remained in position then worms were still present, but if it fell off the child was cured.

Rickets is a disease of infancy which has almost as many folk-cures as whooping-cough. A seventeenth-century prescription consisted in opening a vein in both ears of the child, mixing the blood with lard and rubbing the paste over the child's breast, sides and neck for nine days. Another cure (a favourite in Ireland) was to pass the infant through the split halves of an ash tree. The association of trees with the future health of a child is an almost world-wide belief. Maori families of New Zealand take the umbilical cord of the infant, place it in the ground and plant a sapling over it. As long as the tree continues to thrive so will the child. The custom of planting a tree at birth is found in many parts of Europe, and in some countries there is the belief that the tree must first be split, the child passed through, and the tree then bound up securely. If the binding holds, the child will have good health, but if it splits a life of illness lies ahead.

The urge to protect the newly-born from future illness and misfortunes is deep and powerful, and shows itself in a thousand customs and superstitions propagated by generations of midwives in many countries and communities. One of the oldest superstitions is that it is unlucky for the child to be weighed again after birth until it is twelve months old. Nurses, paediatricians and health-visitors still have to contend with this belief today. It is also believed in some parts of England that the nails of an infant should not be cut for a year, or he will develop a propensity for stealing, while in other areas the right hand of the infant must not be washed for a similar period to ensure that money "sticks" to it. Associated with the cure of many outward signs of illness, or with wounds, is the healing power of human spittle. Birth marks, often said to be in the shape of some object that frightened the mother during pregnancy, can be removed by the mother licking the place for nine days. Perhaps the ancient "kiss the place to make it well" technique used by countless mothers has a practical as well as a psychological application, for spittle certainly appears to have mild curative and antiseptic properties.

Actual bodily harm can be done to children inadvertently by those who have not studied the folklore of infancy sufficiently. For example, stepping over a crawling baby has long been held to stunt its growth. In Italy no child is ever given red shoes to wear, or allowed to eat red fruits such as strawberries or cherries. The effect of this colour on a sensitive infant is to develop unpleasant antisocial behaviour in later life, including bad-tempers and uncontrollable rage. A child's well-being can be measured in several ways, one of the most venerable being the use of a piece of coral tied round the child's neck. If the coral grows pale the infant is about to suffer some ailment, and the coral will not resume its colour until the condition improves. In parts of Britain and America similar reliance is placed on the umbilical cord of the baby, which is carefully kept locked away and consulted from time to time in cases of illness. If the cord remains moist and full the health of the child will not be impaired, but if the cord withers and dries then the illness will be of a serious nature and will not respond to treatment until the condition of the cord improves. This is not the only example in which the body of the child itself is seen to be endowed with some magical property against disease. A footling (a child born feet first) has long been attributed with the power of healing rheumatism, lumbago and similar afflictions. The child only has to trample on the victim for relief to follow! Of particular value in illness is the presence of a child whose mother died while giving birth, and the breath of a posthumous baby has often been used to cure all manner of conditions, and is second only in this capacity to the seventh child of a seventh child. The association of ideas between the innocence of children and their power to avert the influence of evil is seen in many cultures. The Incas of Peru, for example, had enormous faith in the power of blood drawn from between the eyebrows of a five-year-old boy to ward off any and every illness. Most curious is the belief, common in many countries of Europe, that the child will change fundamentally every seven years until it is twenty-one. So strong is this idea that in the nineteenth century many cases were reported of parents refusing treatment for a child suffering from blindness or some crippling deformity, in the belief that it would be automatically cured when the child reached the age of seven, or if not then, at fourteen. Superstition and ignorance such as this has caused untold misery and suffering to many children and it is hard to believe that such ideas persist today. But not all children are protected as assiduously as is intended by these superstitions. The lot of the changeling child was grim indeed in an age when mental retardation was not understood. It was easy for the parents of a deficient child to persuade themselves that it was not really theirs, but had been changed at birth by witches, or more likely, by fairies. There was only one solution. The infant had to be made to suffer so badly that the fairy-mother would take pity on it and rescue it from its fate, bringing back the real child to replace it. Appalling cruelty was often shown to small children in this way.

Many animals, especially the sow, will often ill-treat or even kill one of a litter that is smaller or different from the rest. In some instances it can be traced to the fact that the newborn animal, through some malformation or lack of natural ability, gave physical pain to the mother when feeding, or may have caused her excessive pain during birth. Many animals are quick to recognize this, and the neglect of the new arrival, or its rapid death by the action of the mother, will often result.

In some communities children are ill-treated to propitiate the gods. In times of drought Zulu mothers will take their children and bury them up to their necks in earth, meanwhile indulging in loud wailing and lamentation for the plight of their children. This is supposed to arouse the pity of the gods, who will send rain in order to lessen the suffering of the children. The idea of childish innocence cloaking intense evil has been a popular literary theme. The foremost example of this is the famous Henry James story *The Turn of the Screw* translated, with varying degrees of success, into films, a play and an opera. Students of psychic phenomena have long been of the opinion that the actions of poltergeists are intimately associated with the presence of young children. But one writer, Julian Franklyn, in his *Death by Enchantment*, goes even further. In his opinion there is a direct relationship between the presence of poltergeists and sexual activity in young people. He provides evidence that the actions of a poltergeist can be almost literally "sparked off" when a child masturbates and that the electrical field around a child at such times is greatly intensified. He quotes a case where blue flashes and various electrical disturbances were seen at the upper windows of a girls' school at night when the occupants of the dormitory were supposed to be asleep. In another investigation of a poltergeist on a housing estate in Scotland it was discovered that a nine-year-old boy in the house was regularly masturbating, and when he was discouraged from this activity the actions of the poltergeist ceased immediately. According to this author such odd manifestations are not limited to masturbation on the part of children, and perhaps the most alarming incident quoted is that of the newly-married couple who suffered a powerful electric shock every time they indulged in sex! But even if masturbation does not always result in such startling phenomena, it is common enough to have exercised the minds of many parents and child experts, rarely more so than during the Victorian era. Medical books and "hints to mothers" of this period seem inordinately occupied with this topic, often listed under the heading of "Secret Vice."

A medical manual written in 1884 for the guidance of parents solemnly points out that children who are permitted to "handle themselves" will "become listless and sick, idiotic or even insane, and will develop epileptic fits." Parents of such unfortunates are told to keep their children away from others, or, should this be impossible, always to ensure that they are never left alone. To this is added the somewhat dubious advice that, to effect a cure, the genitals should be frequently washed in cold water and rubbed vigorously with a coarse towel! If "secret vice" should be suspected, the author continues, there should be little difficulty in diagnosing the condition. The signs of self-handling are manifest. The child will be listless, preferring solitude to companionship, and averse to exercise. He (or even she) will have an "averted look," will be nervous, hypochondriachal, restless in sleep, constipated, suffer from constant pain in the back in the mornings and have cold and clammy hands. If a parent is still in doubt, even with these symptoms, there is apparently a final conclusive sign. "The body emits a peculiar disagreeable smell, and there is emaciation."

The connection between masturbation and madness was believed to be close in the nineteenth century. An American doctor writing in 1890 pointed out that of 816 cases of insanity in the New York State Asylum, more than 500 were found to be addicted to masturbation. But there was hope. The cure lay not so much in the hands of the children but in the hands of their parents. Such children should not be punished nor treated as criminals. The answer was in the encouragement of regular habits (though the vice itself could well be classified under this heading) and the immediate stoppage of all "stimulating" foods such as pickles, coffee, spice or pepper well known to heat the blood. Psychologists today might well see in this mal-practice a connection between the penis and a pickled gherkin, but in the nineteenth century science had not progressed to this extent.

In a curiously entitled book *Self-Enervation*, published in America in 1887, a Dr. Eldridge thunders against his own profession for failing to stamp out "secret vice," Parents, too, are accused of neglecting to watch out for signs of this habit, and, as we have seen, the symptoms are described with as much earnestness as parents today are presented with the early symptoms of drug-taking in the young. At all events Victorian writers were more optimistic about self-abuse in children than their modern counterparts are about drugs. Dr. Emma Drake ends on a hopeful note in her treatise on the subject and looks forward to the day when child after child, looking at its parent with clear and candid eyes, will be able to lisp, "Mamma, I am now free from this habit which leads to such untold misery." Any normal child, making this announcement, might well be thought to have left things a little late and to have already succumbed to the mental disturbances fore-cast. Even if the power of the pickle had been overcome in its ability to lead to "secret vice" it still remained a dangerous form of diet for children for other reasons. The Biblical text, "As a man thinketh in his heart, so is he," was quoted to prove this. Plain simple food is recommended for the growing child, lest his tastes become vitiated and his appetite depraved. "The child who swallows spices, condiments, pickles and other irritating or hot substances is certain to think irritating hot thoughts, and to speak hot words."

Such considerations were problems of early childhood, but the feeding habits of the newborn baby were no less important. Bottle-feeding versus breast-feeding has been a topic of controversy for more than a hundred years. Like many other recommendations of the medical profession it suffers from re-thinking every few years, and what may be thought suitable and proper in one generation becomes unhealthy and dangerous in the next, gaining acceptance once more a few years later. The ideal of Victorian motherhood was the breast-fed baby, and the feeding-bottle and teat were abhorred by most doctors, who claimed they led to such afflictions as malformation of the mouth, and digestive troubles. If the mother could not feed her child herself, it was better to hire a wet-nurse than let the child be fed artificially. Copious instructions are given for the choice of such a woman. She should be between twenty and thirty, in perfect health and of sound morals, with "full round breasts" and nipples "erectile and firm."

If one believes the *Household Physician* of 1885, when a girl applied for a position as wet-nurse she was likely to be forced to undergo an examination more suitable for Cruft's or the Smithfield Show. According to the writer, "She should be carefully examined to ensure that she is free from any communicable disease such as consumption or syphilis. For this purpose her teeth, gums, throat, skin and hair should be inspected. Her breasts should be firm, not fat or flabby, and the nipples should be free from fissures. Her milk should be examined, and should be sweetish and blueish-white. On standing it should yield a considerable quantity of cream."

But this was not the end of the ordeal. Her morals and habits were the subject of close scrutiny, as were the morals and habits of her husband. Her general demeanour and temperament was investigated. "Next to the quality of her milk, the quality of her temper is of the highest importance." Needless to say she was strictly forbidden any spirits, beer or porter, though fifty years earlier the enlightened Mrs. Beeton thought otherwise and suggested that the wet-nurse be allowed half a pint of stout mid-morning, a pint of porter with her lunch, a half-pint of stout with her supper and a final pint of porter before going to bed! But the Total Abstinence Movement had scarcely started in Mrs. Beeton's day and there was far less supervision of nurses, wet or dry.

Jane Austen tells how certain women in the village were professional wet-nurses, taking in several children from wealthy families and feeding them all at breast, the parents being allowed to visit two or three times a week. This may have worked well in rural areas, but in town it was dangerous to take such risks. Quite apart from the neglect and hardship which might be suffered by the infant there was, in some cases, a real danger to its life. The lowest form of wet-nurse, who had probably put her own illegitimate offspring on the parish, was not averse to insuring her infant charges, disposing of them and collecting the compensation. The notorious Mrs. Dyer, the Reading baby-farmer who was eventually hanged in 1898, is a well-documented case and was the subject of many broadsheets and ballads. At least one of them may still be heard at London's Players Theatre today:

> *Oh say, have you heard of the famous Mrs. Dyer,*
> *Who at the Old Bailey's awaiting her pay?*
> *In times long ago she'd have burned on the fire*
> *And thus would have perished that wicked old jay!*

Inevitably, "pickles, condiments and cucumbers" were banned to the wet nurse who performed, on the whole, a useful and necessary function. One wonders how any of them passed the test or agreed to the restrictions put on their work, yet the personal columns of Victorian newspapers are sprinkled with offers of "good breast milk" available, with assurances as to the supplier's health and morals. In an age which concerned itself so much with the education of young mothers, it is odd how many of their duties were left to others.

5

Household Cures and
Self-Medication

THE advent of the National Health Service in Britain in 1948 revived many previously-held theories about the effect of a state-subsidized system of free medicine. There was the fear that doctors and hospitals would be swamped by malingerers and the frivolous, that public funds would be wasted on patent or popular remedies, and that those willing to continue paying for treatment would have advantages over those unable to afford it. The *White Paper* of Beveridge in 1942, on the other hand, expressed the hope that such a system would encourage people to consult a doctor more often, and so reduce cases of illness. A *Times* editorial of 1943 predicted that "any health budget will show on the credit side a substantial saving to the nation by the reduction of disease." The patent medicine trade, in particular, feared for its future, for with free advice and prescriptions for all it saw little incentive for the man-in-the-street to go on buying the old proprietary products.

A quarter of a century later we can see the situation in perspective, and judge how many of these fears were justified. There are difficulties at present in obtaining free dental treatment but on the whole the picture has developed differently. People are not less ill, though the pattern of disease has changed, and people have not stopped buying patent medicines.

Few people admit to being in perfect health—in fact only about one in three of the urban population, according to a survey carried out in recent years.* About the same number consider their state of

* *Health and Sickness: the Choice of Treatment* by Wadsworth, Butterfield and Blaney (Tavistock Publications, 1971).

health to be "reasonable" while the rest are certain they are ailing. Even amongst those admitting to reasonable or perfect health, 95 per cent had experienced some minor symptom or complaint during the fourteen days immediately preceding the survey.

From these figures one might expect doctors' surgeries to be even more congested than they are, for even with the prescription charge the National Health Service offers a vast saving to the public in the cost of treatment and medication. In fact the survey, and others conducted since, confirmed what had previously been suspected—that only about one person in four experiencing symptoms or feeling unwell actually seeks medical advice. There are several reasons why three-quarters of the British public still prefers to treat itself at home rather than go to the doctor. There is, and always has been, a corpus of minor ailments that has traditionally responded to home medication. This includes coughs, colds, headaches, constipation and minor digestive disturbances, conditions which many overworked doctors actively discourage from presenting at surgery.

A secondary reason is that though the N.H.S. may theoretically save money it does not save time. Millions of people prefer to treat themselves with a bottle of aspirin or ask the pharmacist to recommend a "tonic" rather than sit for hours in a crowded surgery. The sale of specifics for home medication, though it has changed in nature, continues to increase. In the United Kingdom, for example, 40 per cent of the population have regular recourse to pain-killers, yet only 10 per cent of these do so on medical advice. Again, ointments and medication for the skin are used by millions of people daily, but 4 out of 5 do so without consulting a doctor. In most cases self-medication seems to alleviate the symptoms and may often arrest the progress of the illness. It saves time for the sufferer, allows him to continue at work, and reduces congestion in the surgery.

The kinds of medicine available for use in the home, though greatly changed over the years, can be classified roughly into three types. First are the highly-publicized "patent" medicines in common use, many of which have a tradition of success extending back two hundred years and more. Second come the many chemicals evolved or isolated in laboratories since the eighteenth century and available for purchase over the counter. Quinine is an early example, with aspirin, codeine, magnesium trisilicate phenacetin and caffein as later developments.

Finally there remains the vast range of herbal remedies used for centuries and whose success is based on a mixture of faith, folklore, superstition and science.

Patent Medicines in the Home

From the mid-seventeenth century, druggists, doctors and others with medical knowledge began to market, under their own name, a whole range of cures and medicines. Only rarely did they actually list the ingredients. There was a rough-and-ready system of registration and patent but this did little to protect trade names, and many of the more successful of these proprietary medicines were sold by different people under identical names and in almost identical packs. Needless to say, each manufacturer claimed to be the "original" and warned the public of "inferior substitutes." Daffy's Elixir, for example, first advertised in 1720 as "wonderfully successful in relieving persons afflicted with Stone and Gravel, Dropsy, Surfeits and Gripes," had several competitors. The *London Advertiser* of 29th October, 1743, carried two almost identical advertisements in the same column, one for "Daffy's Elixir" the other for "Dr. Daffy's Elixir." Each claimed to be the genuine product, each claimed that its distinctive trademark was the original, and each warned against counterfeits. In the event it was probably "Daffy's" rather than "Dr. Daffy's" that was genuine, as this was sold by the daughter of the inventor, though she succeeded in confusing the public even more by stating that "Daffy's Elixir is prepared by me, and *no one else* (except by my brother, Anthony Daffy)."

Gravel or stone in the kidney was a scourge from ancient times, and most remedies on the market purported to ease it as a bonus to whatever else they claimed to cure. Popular, too, were the several brands of "female pills" on the market, one of the earliest and most famous being those of Dr. John Hooper. Turlington's Balsam of Life was another favourite, and in 1726 King George I granted a patent for the making of Dr. Bateman's Pectoral Drops.

In 1783, as a direct result of the crippling cost of the long war with the American Colonies, the first tax was imposed on patent medicine.

The product went tax-free only if its formula was disclosed. The medical profession was also concerned with the quality of the drugs used in these 'patents' even if their overall efficacy was not in doubt. In 1864 the first British Pharmacopoeia laid down standards for drugs used, those that conformed having the letters B.P. after the name. But this was only a standard, and did not impose a legal duty on the manufacturer to use such drugs. In the meantime the patent Medicine Stamp still gave the manufacturer the choice of disclosing his formula and not paying tax, or keeping it a secret and putting the government stamp on the bottle. This system did not come to an end until 1941. The presence of the stamp on their products was turned to good account by some manufacturers who, in their publicity, implied that it meant government approval of the contents.

During the nineteenth century the sale of patent medicines reached unprecedented heights in Britain and America. The advertisement pages of newspapers and magazines of a century ago demonstrate the size of the business done. Cures were advertised for every known illness as well as for many unknown ones invented by the manufacturers to worry the public. But the trade faced plenty of opposition, most of it from the medical profession. Doctors were already worried about the increasing tendency of chemists and druggists to diagnose and prescribe rather than refer the patient to a doctor. Manufacturers who disclosed their formulae, and many who did not, found their products listed in publications claiming to "reveal" the ingredients and cost. One such was *Secret Remedies* issued by the British Medical Association itself in an attempt to wean the public away from them. But they did not get very far. Many patent medicines had too much success behind them, and old favourites like Anderson's Pills, first sold in 1630, or Dr. James Fever Powders, dating from 1747, were very difficult to dislodge.

Across the Atlantic the birth of nationhood had fostered a new pride in all things made in America. During the revolutionary war (1776–83) many of the patent medicines imported from England had not been available and American druggists slowly began to evolve their own nostrums to replace them. But again the old remedies died hard and it was more profitable to compound these mixtures in America but to preserve the original English names and packaging.

Empty bottles were imported, filled with ingredients approximating to the original formula, labelled accordingly and provided with a facsimile of the English Government Patent Medicine Stamp. Later, American-made bottles came into use, and even specially-shaped ones like those used for Turlington's Balsam were made. This mixture, incidentally, secured such a grip on the American market that some full bottles

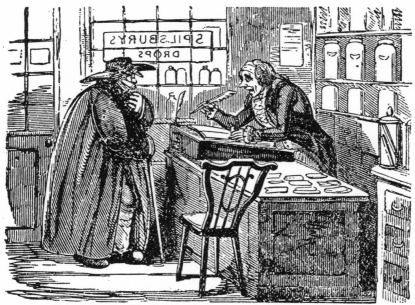

Price defrauding Mr. Spilsbury under the assumed Name of Wilmot.

5 A dispensary in eighteenth century London

were actually found in an Indian burial-chamber, presumably provided to bring solace to the departed in the next world. In 1821 the first professional pharmaceutical body was founded in America, the Philadelphia College of Pharmacy. It is significant that when it published its first book of medical formulae in 1824 the eight medicines listed were the eight most popular English patent medicines! Even when American druggists began to make their own patent nostrums they were reluctant to ascribe them to the New World. One of the earliest, first advertised in the *Boston News-Letter* in 1763, claimed to be an ancient Greek recipe that would "convert a Glass of Water into the Nature and Quality of Asses Milk with the Balsamick Addition."

Gradually American druggists and manufacturers acquired more confidence and new remedies with local names began to appear. Dr. Swayne's Consumption Cure came from Philadelphia, and advertisements appeared for Brandreth's Pills made in Sing-Sing, New York. The *Pennsylvania Gazette* puffed the power of "Widow Read's Ointment for the Itch," though it was doubtful if the good lady paid anything for the publicity. The paper was owned by Benjamin Franklin, and Mrs. Read was his mother-in-law.

By 1804 there were between eighty and ninety American-made patent medicines on the market of which the first actually registered, in 1796, were the Bilious Pills of Samuel Lee, Jun., of Windham, Connecticut. But the greatest and most successful of all medicine-men in America in those years was an Englishman, Thomas Dyott. He had come to America as a youth in 1795 and earned his living as a shoe-black. He was resourceful and imaginative and before long was making his own boot-polish in his lodgings and selling it to his customers. He opened a shop, where he experimented with various chemicals, eventually deciding to launch into the patent medicine business. Gradually he extended his business and began to supply the retail trade, buying and importing his own drugs and chemicals, and later embarking on the manufacture of his own glass bottles. By 1830 he was reputed to be earning 25,000 dollars a year and had incalculable assets in real estate and plant. But a few years later he overreached himself when he started his own bank and crashed disastrously in the financial panic of 1837.

By the 1850s the patent medicine trade had gone full-circle and many American specialties were being exported to Britain. Contrary to the practice of a century before, English manufacturers were now making their own medicines and giving them American names. Ransome's American Pills for Piles was an early example, also said to "Remove Obstruction in the Breast and Lungs and to Promote Free Perspiration." They were made in the Norfolk village of North Walsham but sold extensively through depots in Norwich, York and London.

American doctors and druggists, some genuine but many bogus, sailed from America to England to make their fortunes as Dyott had done the other way a hundred years before. Some founded important and permanent businesses and are still active today. Others came for a quick "kill," offering the latest American treatments for any illness or disease and battening on the belief that anything from America must be the latest and best in its field.

In medicine, as in many other things, the "latest" import from America may well have crossed the Atlantic in the opposite direction many years before, and may be merely returning home. Many British patent medicines, as we have seen, were "acquired" by American druggists while other well-known recipes were presented as new inventions. A curiosity in this field is *opodeldoc*, a liniment made of soap and spirit and described by Paracelsus (1493–1541). In England and Europe it was widely used for rheumatism and muscular pain though it found favour mainly in urban areas. In the 1930s it was still being asked for in many city pharmacies in England and was usually called "dilly-opdock." Under its correct name it had travelled to America where it became a generic term for any embrocation or liniment. In 1820 New England newspapers were carrying advertisements for "J. P. Whitewell's Improved Embrocation or Opodeldoc," while at the same time a certain Dr. Steer urged the customer to ensure that his name alone appeared on the label. Strangely, the word also became associated with American country folk of a certain kind, and travelling players often included a rustic comic described as "an old opodeldoc."

Doan's Back-Ache Pills, a famous seller in Britain and America for more than a century, were first advertised by "Dr." James Doan, a druggist of Kingsville, Ontario, about 1870. He claimed to have acquired the recipe from his aunt, Mary Rogers, a member of "the Canadian Quaker Settlements."

Not only emigrants from Britain spread the patent-medicine gospel overseas. Seamen and ships' doctors played their part too, as happened with Dover's Powders, a mixture of opium and ipecac which still features in most foreign pharmacopoeias to this day. The inventor was the notorious Dr. Thomas Dover, a naval surgeon and native of Bristol, also remembered as one of the party which rescued Alexander Selkirk (the original Robinson Crusoe) from Juan Fernandez in 1708. Thomas Dover also put great faith in mercury as a cure-all, but was realistic enough to advise apothecaries using his remedy that patients should be persuaded to make a will before taking large doses! Just over a century after Dover died in 1741 a Mr. James Crossley Eno was selling his "Fruit Salts" from his pharmacy in Newcastle-on-Tyne. From this busy British seaport merchant seamen spread the fame of Eno's as a laxative and healthful drink, particularly useful in the tropics. The result was a thriving export business for the proprietor upon which he based an enormous advertising campaign for the home market. James Eno is famous in the history of patent-medicines as being the first to use whole-page advertisements in the press, most of which he compiled himself. They are astonishing in their coverage and content, almost every inch of space being taken up with allusions to national events, quotations from Plato, Browning, Thackeray, Pope and others, with often a poem or two included as a bonus ("What nobler aim can Man attain than conquest over human pain?")

As in present-day advertising Eno promised untold advantages and enhanced social prestige from the use of his product. "Riches, Titles, Honour, Power and Worldly Prospects" were to be the rewards of a regular bowel movement induced by Eno's, together with the somewhat mysterious aphorism "A Great Act does not Perish with the Life of him who performs it." Perhaps it is better not to dwell on the implications of this remark.

If Eno's ads were devious and verbose, those of that other redoubtable Victorian advertiser, Thomas Beecham were not. The sheer mass of adverts for "Beecham's" in the nineteenth century made its impact on the social history of the times. They were everywhere—on trams, on trains, on buses, on hoardings, on every bathing-hut and in every newspaper and magazine. Promotional expenditure ran into millions, and Beecham only just failed to get his product emblazoned on the white cliffs of Dover for the benefit of passing mariners. A public outcry had developed against the desecration of the countryside by the enormous proliferation of advertisements. Beecham's great contemporary, Thomas Holloway, had recently succeeded in advertising his ointment on the Pyramids, later going on to endow a complete university for women when he finally retired. This became the Royal Holloway College at Esher, in Surrey, now part of London University. Beecham was remarkable in the ingenuity of his advertising. No new invention or discovery was missed, and was soon put to good use in his ads. Typical was his advertisement of 1880 at a time when the newly-discovered X-rays were hitting the headlines. Holloway pointed out that nobody needed X-rays to discover how many pills were in the box of Beecham's displayed in the chemist's window. All you had to do was to project "£.s.d. rays" across the counter to the value of 1s 1½d, acquire a box, and count them yourself!

Perhaps the most famous story of Beecham advertising concerns the vicar of a poor parish in the East End of London who had insufficient funds to provide his flock with hymn books. Beecham got to hear of it and promptly offered to supply a quantity of books free of charge. The vicar was grateful, but cautious. What did Beecham want in return? Would every other page of the hymn books carry a large advert for the Pills? Beecham assured him that this was not so, and that the hymn books would be completely free of any advertising or commercial blemish. Still slightly suspicious the vicar eventually agreed. In due course the hymn books arrived, and, true to his word, the donor had supplied them with no advertisement or reference to his Pills anywhere in their pages. Or so it seemed. It was not until the carol service later that year that the vicar realized he had been outwitted when to his rage and mortification, he heard his congregation singing:

> *Hark, the herald angels sing*
> *Beechams Pills are just the thing.*
> *For blessed peace and mercy mild—*
> *Two for Mother, one for child!*

The phantom pill merchant had struck again!

Patent-medicine merchants like Holloway and Beecham tower over the others in the annals of the industry. The Victorian public was bombarded and bamboozled by a host of lesser fry promising long life and perfect health in terms which would be considered in the worst taste today. Typical was the Bovril advert of 1890 depicting the Holy Father supping a cup of the healthful beverage. The banner headline announced: 'Two infallible powers—the Pope and Bovril!'

But as well as patent medicines, many "confidential" treatments were also offered to sufferers.

In 1890 an American doctor in practice in Halifax, Yorkshire, made the following announcement: "WEAK MEN suffering from the effect of YOUTHFUL ERRORS, EARLY DECAY, LOSS OF MANHOOD, DISTURBED REST, BLUSHING, LOSS OF FLESH and a general breaking up of physical organization should consult me immediately!" This advertisement also seems to have been an early exercise in media research, for the doctor confined his announcement to the pages of London theatre programmes, no doubt secure in the belief that he was reaching the most dissipated section of the market. Such an advertisement would be both illegal and unethical today.

Three years later, in 1893, the claims made by British medical manufacturers were called to account in the famous case of the Carbolic Smoke Ball Company. The firm had advertised the product as an "infallible cure" for a variety of ailments ranging from whooping cough and snoring to influenza. It was also described as "the new American remedy" but was in fact unknown on that side of the Atlantic. So much confidence did the proprietors have in their Carbolic Smoke Ball that they offered £100 to anyone who contracted influenza after using it. Inevitably a lady used it—and went down with influenza a few days later. She thereupon claimed her £100, but the firm refused to pay. The legal proceedings that followed (Carlill v. The Carbolic Smoke Ball Company, Q.B. 1893) found in favour of the plaintiff and cost the company a great deal more than the £100 originally promised. The Carbolic Smoke Ball continued to sell, even after this set-back, but the claims of the company, and those of many others in the field, became rather more restrained as a result.

Today the content of medical advertising is controlled so rigidly that no manufacturer can claim to "cure" anything. He can "ease" or "bring relief"—he may "alleviate" or "reduce" a condition, but the word "cure" is taboo. In addition there are certain diseases for which treatment can never be advertised to the public, notably cancer, tuberculosis and venereal disease.

Over the years the variety of illnesses afflicting the public has also changed. No longer is there a demand for nostrums to cure "the falling sickness", hysteria or partial paralysis and even the "hot flushes" seem to have paled into insignificance. Yet the British public still spends nearly £80 million a year on patent medicines.

Over-the-counter Drugs and Chemicals

From the early years of the twentieth century public faith in many patent medicines began to wane in the light of new chemical and pharmaceutical knowledge. The Great War (1914–18) had the effect of stimulating research and also resulted in the interchange of ideas and information between various countries. Some new products of the laboratory were released more willingly than others. That most important and successful analgesic, aspirin, was a brand-name of the German firm of Bayer and acquired by the Allies under the Enemy Property Act. Lysol was another invention of this company, also to become part of the armamentarium of the home medicine-chest.

From the 1920s a multiplicity of new and synthetic chemicals became available to the public. Many were compounds of aspirin with other substances such as phenacetin or caffein, and when bought over the counter in bulk from the chemist represented a great saving over the patent equivalent. Many manufacturers, especially those equipped to do serious pharmaceutical research, sold these new products through the chemist under their brand names, but not as patent medicines. One of the most successful and far-seeing was Henry Wellcome, an American pharmacist who came to Britain in 1880 to join his friend Silas Burroughs and found the firm of Burroughs, Wellcome & Co. Wellcome was the first to market a small tablet containing a concentrated and exact amount of drug (previously there had been only capsules, pills, *cachets* and *dragées*) which he sold under the name "Tabloids." The success of this technique was immediate and the name became so popular that in the years that followed Wellcome had to engage in endless litigation to stop other tablet manufacturers from using the word "Tabloid." It is still a registered name and still the property of the company, though no longer used for its products. "Tabloid" today is used mainly to describe a small-format illustrated newspaper, but it remains one of the few proprietary names that has passed into the English language and is found in every dictionary.

Most manufacturers of pills and tablets sold under a brand name charged much more for them than the standard B.P. product obtainable in bulk from the chemist's dispensary. Wellcome was no exception. He justified his higher prices by maintaining that the standard set down by the B.P. was not the highest' obtainable, but only the minimum requirement suitable for human consumption. He claimed that his own standards of manufacture and drug purity were higher, and coined the slogan "B.P. or Better" which the company used for many years to describe its products. This was by no means a frivolous claim and in recent years the standards of the British Pharmacopoeia have been found to admit of extremely wide variations in the way the chemical acts in the body. While a B.P. aspirin, for example, must contain five grains of acetylsalicilic acid, there is no stipulation regarding the mass of the tablet in which it is contained. This may be made of a variety of substances, some extremely soluble but others less so. The solubility of the tablet has a direct bearing on the speed with which the chemical is released in the body, and therefore on the rapidity with which it acts and brings relief, a fact noted by two young Australian chemists in the 1920s when they marketed their own brand of aspirin and called it Aspro. More recently the use of digitalis extract, first isolated by Wellcome and sold under the Tabloid banner as Digoxin, has received a good deal of publicity. Here it was discovered that improved methods of manufacture actually speeded up the metabolism of digoxin in the body, creating problems for doctors in the treatment of the young and the very old, both categories being notoriously sensitive to any variation in dosage.

It is now realized that the overall action of a drug in its passage through the body is conditioned by several factors. The presence or absence of food in the stomach, for example, may have a marked effect not only on the speed of metabolism of the substance but on its chemical structure. For this reason at least one American pharmaceutical company is engaged, not in the evolution and discovery of new drugs, but in new methods of administering existing drugs to the patient. The object is to find techniques to bring the drug into direct contact with the affected organ, either by absorption through the skin or by the use of "micro-capsules" of highly-concentrated chemical that can be inserted into the body where the capsule will dissolve and release the drug on the site. It is possible that one of the first applications of this technique will be in the field of contraception, where the placement of a micro-encapsulated quantity of hormone direct in the uterus will afford protection against conception for up to a year. When used in combination with electronic sensors these new techniques become even more interesting. Experiments with insulin show that the diabetic of the future may no longer have to inject himself several times a day. A micro-encapsulated quantity of highly concentrated insulin will be placed in the body, together with a minute electronic sensor rather smaller than the electronic pacemakers at present used for the heart. When the level of insulin in the blood drops below a pre-determined point this will be noted by the sensor which will automatically release a fresh amount of the drug into the system. It is possible that the daily injection of insulin will be replaced by a minor surgical operation to insert a micro-capsule and sensor every three or four years. Though we may marvel at such techniques and applaud those who have evolved them, the unfortunate fact remains that these are still only symptomatic cures, and we are only a little nearer to finding the basic cause of insulin deficiency, the symptoms of which were described three thousand years ago in an Egyptian manuscript. We should not wonder that, despite modern research, many ordinary people the world over still cling tenaciously to the herbal remedies and superstitions of their forefathers.

Before going on to deal with herbal remedies let us look at one further aspect of self-medication that receives little publicity. This is the habit of seeking advice from the dispensing chemist for minor ailments as an alternative to visiting the doctor. Once, the pharmacist would "make-up" a bottle of mixture or an ointment for the customer tailor-made to his requirements, drawing on his extensive knowledge of drugs and their uses. Today, though many members of the public continue to seek his advice, he is more likely to recommend a proprietary product or a ready-made remedy such as Gees Linctus or a bottle of kaolin-and-morphine mixture, for the enormous volume of National Health Service prescriptions flowing from the surgeries gives him less time for dealing with individual requirements. In some ways this is a pity, for the pharmacist, by virtue of his long training and high academic qualifications, has a far greater knowledge of the action of drugs than most doctors. It is sad, too, that so much of the pharmacist's time should be spent trying to rectify errors made by doctors on prescriptions, and in trying to decipher their handwriting. With the multiplicity of ethical products available (some three thousand in all), many with similar-sounding names, a badly-written or unclear prescription could easily result in the patient being given the wrong medicine. The notorious illegibility of doctors' handwriting is no longer a music-hall joke. It is a serious matter that can put the patient at risk. Should this happen the blame is more likely to fall on the pharmacist for failing to read the prescription correctly than on the doctor for his failure to write it accurately or clearly. That the situation rarely arises is due in no small measure to the vigilance of the pharmacist, who must constantly check-back with the doctor to ensure that he really means what he has written. A prescription for a child, for example, may call for an adult dose of the medicine. This *may* be intentional, but might equally be a mistake on the part of the doctor, brought about by working under pressure. It could also be caused by the pernicious habit of allowing young and untrained receptionists to complete the prescription on a blank form previously signed by the doctor. This sometimes happens when the patient contacts the surgery for a "repeat" prescription in the absence of the doctor. Though the practice is frowned upon by the British Medical Association it unfortunately continues, as any retail pharmacist will testify. Further delays and inconvenience to the patient are often caused by the doctor failing to say how much medication is to be dispensed, or by failing to specify the dosage. The fact that the doctor has already told the patient how to take the medicine is often the reason for not putting this information on the prescription. Yet a survey has shown that more than 30 per cent of those receiving instructions on dosage in the surgery either failed to understand them or forgot them by the time they reached the pharmacy.

The situation may be different in other countries where doctors and pharmacists are less hard-pressed, but in Britain it certainly adds tremendously to the responsibilities of the pharmacist, already forced to work longer hours than most of his customers and often for less money. It may also be the reason why fewer and fewer pharmacists are entering the profession, and of those that do fewer and fewer are willing to engage in the retail side of the business. The result is that in Britain the number of retail pharmacies is dropping by about two hundred every year, a situation that will do untold harm to the best state medical service yet devised.

6

Herbal Remedies

IN the grounds of Hardwick Hall, the fine Tudor property in Derbyshire, is a large herb garden containing more than a hundred plants, most of which are recommended for the cure of one or more ailments. Yet these are only a fraction of the total number of plants used medicinally. Hardwick is one of the few remaining examples of the many physic-gardens that existed in town and country in the sixteenth and seventeenth centuries.

The range of herbal remedies is vast. Indeed, it has been said that there is a plant to cure every known disease—the only problem is finding it! Since man first noticed that sick animals instinctively sought out certain roots and herbs the search has continued for plants to benefit mankind. The Greeks and Romans, and before them the Chinese, all had recourse to such remedies and have left records of the diseases they treated. It is not always easy to identify the plant concerned and in many cases their claims are hard to believe. In medieval Europe, for example, a plant known as the springwort was said to have the power of discovering hidden treasure, to open locks and to make the possessor invisible! Unfortunately, the identity of this plant remains obscure, and so the claims made for it cannot be tested. Yet full instructions are given for collecting springwort. Simply block up a cuckoo's nest, spread a red rag below it, and await events. The cuckoo, unable to enter the nest, will fly away to collect a sprig of springwort which it will then hold against the obstruction in the nest. The nest will open magically, and the springwort will fall on to the red rag. It was essential to catch it before it actually reached the ground. To complicate matters still more, the cuckoo has no nest of its own, but uses those of other birds, a fact apparently overlooked by the ancient writers of herbals.

Less fanciful, and obviously based on long experiment and acute observation, are the ancient Chinese herbal remedies of four thousand years ago. One such was the use of the juice of a certain Chinese fir for the treatment of asthma and bronchitis. Not until 1878 was it discovered that this juice contains the alkaloid ephedrine, today almost indispensable in the treatment of pulmonary disorders.

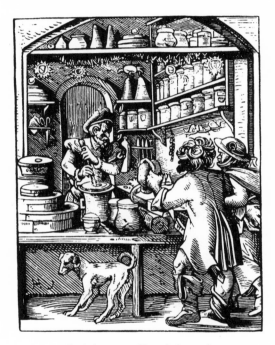

6 A late medieval druggist

In Europe the secrets of the Orient were to remain hidden for many centuries, and much of the medical lore of the Greeks and Romans was forgotten. The medical properties of plants were listed in various herbals from the thirteenth century onward, but not until the great voyages of exploration in the fifteenth and sixteenth centuries, when new and wonderful plants were brought back to Europe, was the true extent of herbal cures first appreciated. Most of the herbals that form the basis of modern plant remedies date from this period.

75

The introduction of printing during the Renaissance also allowed crude illustrations of the plants to be used, making identification easier. Most of the material was from ancient sources and hand-written Latin manuscripts, and the first authentic printed English herbal was that of John Banckes, which appeared in 1525. In 1550 an English physician, Anthony Askham, printed an enlarged version of the Banckes herbal and for the first time attributed the action of herbs to the influence of astrology "declaring what Herbes hath influence of certain Sterres."

In 1526 *The Great Herbal* had been printed, a translation of the French *Le Grand Herbier*, which not only described and illustrated a wide variety of medicinal plants but also included animal and mineral materia medica then in fashion. By the end of the sixteenth century many new drugs and plants were coming into use, brought from the Americas by European explorers. Guaicum, known as *Lignum vitae*, came from South America and the West Indies and the expressed juice of the tree as a cure for syphilis remained in use all over Europe for many centuries to follow. Logwood, balsam of tolu for coughs, sarsaparilla and Winter's bark were all added to the herbals of the day, and in many cases attempts were made to grow the plants in this country.

Many of the great herbalists are still remembered and their writings still used. Probably the greatest authority was John Gerard, born in 1542 in Cheshire and for twenty years head gardener to the powerful Cecil family during the reign of Queen Elizabeth I. He was a member of the company of Barber-Surgeons and in 1597 published his great *Herbal* in three volumes. Twenty years after his death it was enlarged and edited by Thomas Johnson and it is this edition that is normally used today.

A rather more colourful and flamboyant figure was Nicholas Culpeper (1616–54), astrologer and physician in the City of London. The son of a clergyman, he had studied at Cambridge and was proficient in Latin and Greek. His first herbal, called *A Physical Directory* was published in 1649 and immediately created trouble for the author. In the first place it was a translation of the *Pharmacopoeia* of the College of Physicians undertaken without their permission; secondly it contained many acid criticisms of the medical theories held by the

College; and thirdly it was the first herbal to repeat the earlier contentions of Thomas Johnson that astrology had an influence on the healing power of herbs. The College of Physicians was quick to castigate Culpeper and defend itself. It began by severely censuring him for plagiarizing their own publication, showered ridicule on his astrological theories and ended by describing him as "a drunk and a lecher." As so often happens when a work creates dissension and dispute the resultant publicity brought Culpeper to the attention of a wide and international public and ensured that his *Herbal* should be read and studied for the next three hundred years.

Another famous herbalist was John Tradescant, head gardener to King Charles I. Tradescant travelled widely in North Africa, and in his physic-garden in South Lambeth cultivated for the first time many exotic plants unfamiliar to English eyes. John Parkinson (1567–1650) was another great herbalist, traveller and writer with a flair for publicity. He called his *Herbal* of 1629 "Paradisi-in-Sole" a Latin pun on the name Park-in-Sun, and in the same year was appointed Botanist Royal to King Charles I.

The herbals and treatises written by these men, and many others, still included much superstition and "magic" and everywhere the long-standing fear of witchcraft is apparent. The great scientific societies of the day, notably the Royal Society, did much to dispel these old beliefs, and the medical societies in particular studied the properties of plants and herbs with the aid of their own physic-gardens. In London the Society of Apothecaries had their garden in Swan Walk, Chelsea, from 1673 and at Oxford the University established a garden opposite Magdalen Bridge. Both these herb gardens still exist and may be visited. The Chelsea Physic Garden is now under the control of the Royal Botanical Society.

Many plants were known by experience to be useful in alleviating certain symptoms. Others however were thought to be of value merely because they seemed to have some affinity to the symptoms. The diuretic action of the dandelion, for example, was widely used to treat kidney and liver disorders, and was also thought to impart great physical strength. But the little eye-bright was used as a cure for failing eye-sight merely on account of the resemblance of the flower to the human eye, just as the Adder's Tongue Fern, because of its shape, was said to be a specific for snake-bite and to cure soreness in the tongue.

The theory that a disease could be treated by a plant that in some way resembled the symptoms of the patient is an ancient one. In the first century A.D. Diocorides speaks highly of the red juice of the alkanet as an antidote to inflammation of the skin. Some fifteen hundred years later Queen Elizabeth I was employing the same principle when she ordered her bedroom to be hung with red while she was suffering from smallpox.

But most herbal remedies were based on more rational thinking than this. They were also based on a long history of usage and effectiveness. The belladonna plant was used in ancient Mesopotamia to combat bladder spasms, coughs and asthma, while cannabis was employed to relieve pain, and to treat rheumatism and cure insomnia.

In the first years of the Christian era the important Indian medical treatise, the *Charaka Samhita*, already listed more than five hundred herbal drugs, the bulk of which had been known for centuries. Indian doctors had used one particular plant for a wide range of ailments including blood-pressure, colic, headache and nervous disorders. Identified by the German physician and botanist Leonard Rauwolff in 1558, the plant is now known as Rauwolfia. Its various alkaloids are widely used in medicine today. The narcotic mescalin is now known to be the active ingredient of the peyote plant of Mexico, long used by the Aztecs as an anti-depressant and as a means of combating fear, thirst and hunger. It was also said to confer the power of foresight.

Compared with the ancient medical and herbal traditions of the Chinese, Greeks and Romans, or with the exotic products of the forests of Latin America, herbal lore in Europe seems comparatively modern and simple. It was reinforced by the new drugs such as cocoa beans (chocolate was first used as medicine), sarsaparilla and tobacco, the latter described by Christopher Columbus as "effective as a medicine but highly intoxicating." But in most cases the newly-discovered plants had to await the attention of the analysts and pharmacists before their value could be assessed and their use regulated. In the meantime the herbs found near at hand continued to be used, and an ordinary cottage garden contained the means of dealing with virtually any disorder. That there was little logic in many forms of treatment hardly mattered. Faith plays a major part in any curative process, and faith in a herb or plant was likely to effect a cure even if there were no scientific foundation for its action. In modern medical research it is common practice, when testing a new drug, to give a proportion of the patients a placebo—a substance that the patient thinks is the new treatment, but in fact is an inert substance that does nothing at all. Significantly, a percentage of patients taking the placebo always insist that their symptoms are reduced and that their condition has improved. The round mint, so useful in cookery, was used for treating "the languor following epileptic fits." Pennyroyal was popular as a "medicinal" tea and Pliny awarded it the additional bonus of driving away fleas.

Many an old cottager no doubt ensured that he had adequate supplies of Sweet Cicely in his garden, for this was reputed to "increase the lust and strength of the old." Orris root, used by the Greeks and Romans, was popular for bronchitis and dropsy, and wormwood, the active ingredient of which is used in the preparation of absinthe, was highly-prized as an antidote for worms and as a digestive. Foxgloves were used in cases of weak or "tired" heart long before the action of digitalis was discovered, and the juice of onions was considered essential to cure a cough or bronchitis centuries before its use in various patent medicines. In Eastern Europe and in Russia both onion and garlic were used as "sympathetic" remedies, a dried segment of either being worn next to the skin to avoid a heart-attack. Eating raw onions was considered a sure cure for epilepsy.

Contrary to popular belief, the treatment of disease does not progress in an orderly manner as new medicines are discovered. There are fashions in medicine as in anything else, and the treatment for any illness varies enormously from country to country. The advisability of taking exercise in arthritis is argued back-and-forth by physicians alleged to be specialists in their field. In Britain the medical profession concerns itself greatly with diseases of the chest and muscular conditions, whilst in France doctors pay more attention to diagnosing cirrhosis of the liver and to the malfunction of the vascular system. The use of certain drugs or plants in the treatment of illness also tends to suffer from the vagaries of fashion, a striking example being the great "rhubarb mania" that swept across Europe in the eighteenth century.

Rhubarb had been known in Europe from Roman times and was considered one of the most valuable of all vegetables as a cure for almost all diseases. Originally from Korea via China, it was available in only minute quantities and came to Europe by way of Bokhara in Central Asia and the Black Sea. The cost was understandably high, and in the seventeenth century was three times the price of opium, four times that of saffron and ten times that of cinnamon. As the result of an increasing demand for this wonder-plant the Royal Society of Arts in Britain appointed a special committee in 1763 "to pursue the requisite measures for introducing the culture of pure rhubarb." One of the difficulties was that though various rhubarb seeds and plants had reached England, only one variety, the "true" Shensi rhubarb, was effective medicinally.

Success was finally achieved through the agency of Alexander Dick, then president of the Royal College of Physicians in Edinburgh, whose brother-in-law, by a happy chance, was British Resident at the Tsar's court at St. Petersburg. After much conniving and subterfuge involving the Tsar himself and his private physician, who also happened to be English, a box of "true" rhubarb seeds was smuggled out of China through the Russian medical services in Asia. They were planted in the Imperial Botanical gardens at St. Petersburg, and when the Tsar's doctor returned to England he brought with him a tray of those same "true" seeds for distribution to the Royal Society. A well-known Scottish landowner, James English, succeeded in cultivating the seeds and produced mature plants for the inspection of the Society. This august body expressed itself satisfied, granted a gold medal to Alexander Dick and James English for their initiative, and announced the award of a similar medal annually for whoever could grow the most rhubarb plants in Britain.

During the next twenty-five years the medal was won twenty times. The most expert planter of all was a chemist, Thomas Jones, who, on a plot of ground he rented at Enfield, Middlesex, grew more and more rhubarb until in 1797 he had no less than five thousand plants waving in the breeze. By this time the Royal Society was in no doubt that true rhubarb had arrived in Britain and had come to stay, and made a final and somewhat desperate payment to Jones of thirty guineas in token of his outstanding work. But Jones was not to be stopped, and by 1800 had planted another four thousand roots. Fortunately most of the larger hospitals had faith in the plant, and rhubarb was in daily use at Guy's, St. Bartholomew's, St. Thomas's and many other hospitals both in London and the provinces. Today the mind boggles at the employment of so much rhubarb, but the Society was able to announce that in 1801 the total value of the rhubarb market was £200,000. Jones later turned his attention to another crop encouraged by the Royal Society, this time the cultivation of poppies for the production of opium. He produced 21 pounds of the drug from five acres of poppies and was awarded fifty guineas as a result. But though he had proved it could be produced commercially, the collection of the latex from the poppies was no easy thing, and the plants were highly sensitive to wind and rain. Jones returned to his rhubarb.

Today few medicinal herbs are grown in cottage gardens, nor do the learned societies offer many prizes for their cultivation. But herbal cures are big business, with some twent-five commercial firms engaged in the manufacture and supply of packeted herbs. An even larger number of firms concerns itself with the manufacture of natural health foods, ranging from such surprising fruits as "unsophisticated Afghanistan apricots" to the homely kelp or bladderwrack of the seashore. Specialist magazines and periodicals promise glowing health and long life to those willing to adopt "Nature's way." A feature of these publications is the constant criticism of the medical profession for its failure to solve the problems of disease and provide permanent cures. Writing in the magazine *Health for All* in 1973 an American stated categorically that "many thousands of sick people are slaughtered annually in the quiet of the sickroom and then are said to have died because their physicians could not save them." His argument—and it is not a new one—is that modern medicine can only relieve symptoms, and that the long-term use of many substances is more dangerous than the illness they are intended to relieve. Those who study the pages of the health magazines are offered every kind of advice on exercise and diet to ensure perfect health. If they followed these precepts, they would presumably never suffer from anything at all. Both editorial columns and advertisement pages promise relief for almost every known condition, and one must assume that the readership is composed of those less healthy than most. They may also be more gullible, for many of the conditions described and the benefits promised are decidedly vague. Claims that a certain herb (in this case, borage) will "improve the emotional state and give joy to life" abound, while another decoction is described as being "a natural strengthening and building-up medicine." An advertisement for a commercial pack of beetroot juice appears to hark back to the ancient theory of like curing like in its statement that "the natural colouring of the beetroot closely resembles haemoglobin and therefore helps in the regeneration of the bloodstream." One wonders how many readers are in a position to decide if their bloodstream needs "regenerating"? In the same issue an editorial advises readers to drink hawthorn tea to reduce the pulse-rate, while later on we are told that "we should all try a course of magnesium and calcium supplementation to see if we have any deficiency." Most surprising are some of the claims made for grapes. According to an announcement in the magazine *Prevention* a simple diet of grapes has been of value in the treatment of rheumatism, arthritis, kidney complaints, stomach ulcers, migraine, alcoholism and mental instability. With the "nature cure" industry geared either to the relief of symptoms or to protecting the reader from illnesses that he is probably never likely to suffer from, it is no surprise that business is booming. Thousands of people who claim to distrust doctors and begrudge the cost of medical insurance cheerfully spend their hard-earned money on products of unspecified content, products which promise only to "revitalize the bloodstream, give sparkle to the eye, colour to the lips and spring to the step." Curiously enough, few people who swallow either these tonics or their descriptions seem to prove their efficacy. Anyone living on a diet of soya-beans and seaweed could hardly be expected to be full of *joie-de-vivre*. Market research comes to the aid of the herbal advertiser as much as it does to any form of consumer selling, and no doubt the industry is acting wisely when it spends such fortunes on advertising cures for "nervous exhaustion, tension, emotional instability and stress." Perhaps the most honest advice is unwittingly provided in the title of a book written by John B. Lust, a well-known advocate of "natural" foods. It is called *Drink Your Troubles Away.*

Despite the fanciful claims of some commercial herbal specialists, there is no doubt that hundreds of plants do give at least symptomatic relief in many complaints. This is the basis of modern pharmacology. It is hard to see why, when the active ingredient of a plant is isolated and standardized in the laboratory, it should immediately become the "harmful drug" so hated by the herbalists. It is surely better for the elderly cardiac patient to receive a controlled quantity of digoxin prescribed by his doctor than to try and survive on a daily intake of a decoction of foxgloves. It is the chemicals present in plants and herbs that produce their action on the body. Just how much of a chemical is present, and how much good it does, varies greatly and depends on the method of cultivation, time of harvesting and later treatment such as drying, packaging and storing. Many of today's "ethical" or prescription drugs are those self-same chemicals extracted or manufactured under strict laboratory conditions instead of in the plant, and so are much purer and allow more certainty of action. Yet there has always been a resistance to prescribed medicine and a tendency to go back to "simples" and herbal cures. John Wesley himself was an outspoken champion of "natural" methods of healing. In 1747 he published his own medical text-book, the *Primitive Physick: Or an Easy and Natural Method of Curing most Diseases.* In it, he soon makes clear his views on orthodox medicine : "And against the greater part of these medicines there is a further Objection : They consist of too many Ingredients. This Common Method of compounding and decompounding medicines can never be reconciled with Common Sense. Experience shows that One Thing will cure most disorders at least as twenty put together. Then why do you add the other nineteen? Only to swell the Apothecary's bill : Nay, possibly on purpose to prolong the Distemper, that the Doctor and he may divide the Spoil."

Many of Wesley's remedies are simple, safe and sound and are an accepted part of home medication to this day. Others, however, are a little surprising, such as his treatment for consumption. This consists of "cutting a little turf of fresh earth, lying down and breathing into the hole a quarter of an hour." In the advanced stages of this disease he recommends the even more remarkable expedient of "sucking a healthy woman daily" and claims his father was cured by this means. Strangely enough, modern research into vitamins indicates that this treatment may not be as nonsensical as it sounds. Breast milk is a rich source of vitamin C (cows' milk contains virtually none) and vitamin C has been shown to have some action against the tubercle bacillus.

From the pages of Wesley, from the writings of the great herbalists and even from such amateurs as Hannah Glasse, whose cookery book of 1745 included many prescriptions, a solid core of herbal remedies persists and is constantly regurgitated in later writings.

Any attempt to describe them all would be impossible. Instead details are given below of some which are well-known, and whose action in the treatment of various diseases seems to have stood the test of time.

ANGELICA
For the treatment of coughs, colds and pleurisy. An ingredient of Vermouth and Chartreuse.

BROOM
Used in the treatment of kidney and bladder infections.

CELANDINE
An ancient remedy for jaundice, ringworm and haemorrhoids. Also, one of the many remedies for warts.

COLTSFOOT
One of the oldest specifics for coughs and chest complaints.

DANDELION
Used for kidney and liver disorders. Its French name *pis-en-lit* (piss-in-bed) refers to its action as a diuretic.

DOCK
The root or leaves of the dock are often used in country districts to cure skin rashes and as an antidote to stinging by nettles.

GERMANDER
Said to be useful for treating rheumatism and gout.

HYSSOP

The green tops are infused for use in the treatment of stomach complaints, rheumatism and chest troubles. Used in the manufacture of Benedictine, Chartreuse and many liqueurs.

IVY

Juice from the plant sniffed up the nose was said to cure heavy catarrh and head colds. An infusion made from the leaves was used for sore eyes and for skin infections, and a wreath of ivy was worn on the head to stop baldness!

JUNIPER

Smoke from burning juniper wood was long held by the ancients to dispel infection. The oil of the plant has been used for dropsy, liver troubles and rheumatism, and it is still extensively used as an antidote to back-ache.

LILY OF THE VALLEY

Believed at one time to be of value in heart conditions. Culpeper credits it with the power of restoring speech.

LOOSESTRIFE

As a haemostatic to check bleeding from wounds and popular as a gargle for sore throat.

MALE FERN

The extracted juice of the root is still used to eliminate tapeworms.

MARIGOLD

A plant with a multiplicity of uses including the treatment of bee stings, ague, fever, depression, noises in the head, and inflammation of the eyes.

MARSHMALLOW

Used for bronchitis and coughs and sometimes for bladder disorders. The root is used as a poultice.

MISTLETOE

The "golden bough" of the ancients, associated with many super-stitions and beliefs in many countries. Medically it was thought to be of value in various nervous disorders including St. Vitus' Dance, and was also used for heart troubles, snake-bites, epilepsy, tooth-ache and many other ailments. Not surprisingly it was known as All-Heal and in addition was reputed to be an antidote for all poisons, to induce fertility in women, and to destroy aggressive instincts in men.

MOTHERWORT

As the name implies it was widely used in the treatment of female disorders. Its botanical name (*Leonorus cardiaca*) gives a hint of its former use in heart disease, and it was often prescribed by herbalists for nervous conditions.

MUGWORT

An ancient and curious belief going back to Pliny is that the juice of the plant will prevent exhaustion on a long journey. The leaves, when worn in the shoes, enabled the wearer to walk forty miles "and not be weary," according to a seventeenth-century herbalist. It was also used for failing sight and to counteract the effects of sunstroke.

NETTLES

An important ingredient of herbal remedies for "cleansing" the blood probably due to the high chlorophyll content. It is also still used to stop nose-bleeding and was considered essential for dealing with what seems to have been the remarkably high incidence of bites from mad dogs in Tudor times and later.

PARSLEY

An ancient specific for kidney disease. To chew the leaves is still considered a means of warding off rheumatism, but perhaps its most valuable attribute, if true, is the capacity to "help men with weyke braynes to beare drinke better."

PERIWINKLE

The leaves are still occasionally used to ease the pains of cramp and boils, and if chewed are said to stop toothache. Culpeper notes that if the leaves are eaten by man and wife together the result will be "to cause love between them."

ROSEMARY

According to the English version of the *Grete Herball* "for weyknesse of ye brayne."

SARSAPARILLA
Much valued as a blood-cleanser.

THYME
Has been used in the treatment of whooping-cough due to its active ingredient, thymol.

VALERIAN
Infusion of valerian is still prescribed as a tranquillizer in nervous troubles often in combination with a bromide.

VERVAIN
Once known as the Holy Herb, this plant comes into the category of the "all-heals" and has been mentioned as beneficial in the treatment of more than thirty complaints. It has long been used for stone in the bladder (the name derives from the Celtic *fer*, to drive away, and *faen*, a stone) and was reputed to cure the King's Evil (scrofula). It was said to have been found growing on Calvary and to have been used to staunch Our Lord's wounds. Because of this it was held to be a specific against bleeding and good for the healing of every kind of wound.

In most countries in the west herbal remedies are considered to be strictly the province of folk-medicine; there is little contact between herbalists and those who practice conventional medicine. This is not so in eastern countries. In China and Japan the two forms of therapy go hand-in-hand, each an integral part of the other. In Japan the technical medical journals carry advertisements for the most sophisticated products of modern pharmaceutical research side-by-side with those for ancient Chinese and Japanese herbal remedies, many of them still prescribed by the doctors. It is therefore no surprise to find that the giant Japanese state-owned Takeda Chemical Company has established, at Kyoto, one of the world's largest herb gardens. Here some four thousand species of plant, mostly medicinal, are grown under near-perfect conditions by a team of research workers. It is interesting, too, that the herb garden is part of Takeda's Research and Development section, for its function is to develop techniques by which the active ingredient of the plant can be made constant and not subject to the wide variations that occur when the plant

is growing in its wild state. At Kyoto there is an unceasing pro-
gramme of cultivation, extraction and assay of herbs and plants
honoured by centuries of usage as folk medicines. Since 1953, for
example, there has been continuing research on the humble rhubarb
so that crops can now be grown not only with a high and predictable
chemical content but also in such a way that many of the unwanted
side-effects of the active ingredient are eliminated. Research is carried
on with such ancient oriental roots as Coptis and Ginseng, the second
of which has only become popular in the west two hundred years
after the original description of its medicinal properties by the Jesuit
missionary, Father Jartoux, in 1711.

Garlic is another plant now undergoing intensive study. Recent
research has contributed greatly to the synthesis of thiamin and
various vitamin-B derivatives. A secondary function of the Kyoto
herb gardens is to test the various products of the parent company
in the ceaseless fight against plant parasites and weeds, and as general
fertilizing agents.

In India, China and Japan, it is realized that modern medicine
and ancient herbal remedies can benefit each other and promote the
well-being of mankind. Traditional herbs can still be the source
of new discoveries in the field of organic chemistry, while modern
laboratory techniques ensure that ancient plant remedies, popular for
centuries, may be used with complete confidence. It is a pity that
more western herbalists do not conduct their business in this precise
and scientific way, instead of making vague and highly fanciful
claims, which has damaged the prestige of their ancient calling.

7

Quacks and their Cures

JOHN WESLEY and others believed that God had provided a plant
to cure every ailment. But herbal remedies were not always as successful as people hoped. Nor, in earlier times, were the services of physicians easily available to ordinary people. Medicine was largely in the
hands of the monks who often limited treatment to those who could
afford their high fees. In 1130 the Council of Clermont, seeking to
discourage clerics from acquiring worldly wealth, forced them to
treat the poor free of charge. The scheme was not altogether successful and by the end of the thirteenth century the Vatican had to forbid
all priests to practise medicine or even to be present at operations.
The way was therefore opened to many amateurs and quacks. Though
the Church forbade its own clergy to practice medicine it still tried
to control the laity in this respect. In England Henry VIII made it
illegal for anyone to cure the sick or diagnose disease without a
licence from the Bishop of London or the Dean of St. Paul's. In
1504, five years before Henry came to the throne, the ancient association of barbers and surgeons had formed their own professional company and allowed only their own members to practise "barbery,
shavery, surgery and the letting of blood" within the City of London.
In 1518 Henry VIII granted a Charter to another branch of medicine,
the College of Physicians, who also made it illegal for any but their
own members to deal in "physick" within seven miles of London. In
other towns and cities local branches of both the Barber-Surgeons and
Physicians attempted to impose similar restrictions locally, and membership of either association called for the passing of examinations
before registration.

In the same way as the barbers and surgeons were united (the red

and white pole of the modern barber represents the blood and band-
age of the barber-surgeon to this day) so the apothecaries were associated with the grocers. This is not as illogical as it might appear, for
the business of apothecary had developed from those members of
the powerful Grocers' Company who specialized in the import of
foreign drugs and spices.

The Apothecaries, like the Surgeons and Physicians, wanted to
became a Company in their own right and to separate from the
Grocers, whom they considered merely as tradesmen. But in their case
it was not so easy, and it was not until 1617 that James I granted
them their charter despite the fears of the Physicians that the Apothecaries might encroach upon their own function—a fear that later
proved to be well-founded.

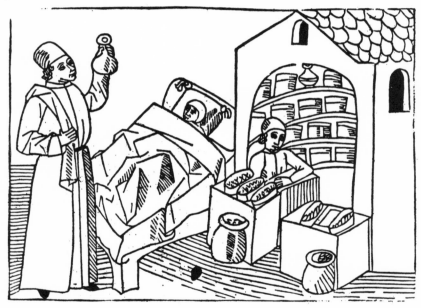

7 A medieval hospital and dispensary

Not only did the physicians face competition from the apothecaries,
but after the Restoration of Charles II in 1660, they faced it from an
army of mountebanks, quacks and swindlers who flocked to England
in his wake. They came from France, Germany, Holland and Italy,

all of them looking upon England as virgin territory in which to test their skills, with many claiming to have received royal patronage from Charles during his years of exile. They did not have it all their own way. The laxity of life after the rigours of the Commonwealth period encouraged many English quacks to come into the open and practice more blatantly than anyone had done for a hundred years. They were soon joined by others from Scotland and Ireland, and by the mid-eighteenth century the quack-doctor in England had achieved a notoriety and position that was never to be surpassed. Not for nothing is this era described as "the golden age of quackery," and many were the colourful and bizarre practitioners who amassed fortunes in those years. They were helped by the incredible gullibility of the public and the comparative ease with which licences could be had from the bishops. The hallmark of the quack, and the reason he is so called, lies in the loud and strident voice with which he proclaims the value of his cures. One early impostor was Thomas Saffold, who obtained his licence from the Bishop of London in 1674, and advertised in verse beginning:

It's Saffold's Pills, much better than the rest,
Deservedly have got the name of Best.

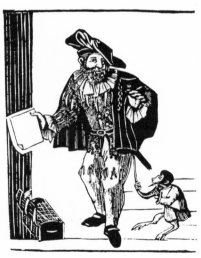

8 A quack at the fair

Another seventeenth-century impostor was the notorious Dr. Case who claimed to cure :

> *The Cramp, the Stitch,*
> *The Squirt, the Itch,*
> *The Gout, the Stone, the Pox;*
> *The Mulligrubs,*
> *The Bonny Scrubs*
> *And all Pandora's Box.*

Case was honest, or impudent, enough to end his doggerel with the lines :

> *Read judge and try*
> *And if you Die*
> *Never believe me more!*

Not content with the multiplicity of known ailments waiting to be cured many quacks invented others of their own, safe in the knowledge that nobody else could treat them ! A seventeenth-century booklet purporting to be a treatise on female disorders undertook to cure "The Glimm'ning of the Gizzard, the Quavering of the Kidneys and the Wambling Trot."

One of the most successful quacks was William Read of Aberdeen, an uneducated tailor who could scarcely read or write. He set up as an itinerant oculist, and after travelling widely in the north of England and Ireland came to London in 1700. Here he gained a certain amount of publicity by offering free treatment to any soldier who had served with Marlborough in the French wars. He came to the notice of Queen Anne, herself a permanent victim of weak eyes, who awarded him a knighthood in 1705, to the intense annoyance of the medical profession. As Sir William Read he was accepted in society, if not by the physicians, and became an intimate of both John Addison and Jonathan Swift. When Read died in 1715, a year after the Queen, his wife tried to continue his work at Court, but the new King, George I, did not approve of her and she was pensioned off : not, it seems, because of her lack of experience or knowledge, for King George appointed an even greater charlatan as Royal Oculist, a man called Roger Grant, a one-eyed illiterate cobbler who had served in the army before trying his luck as an Anabaptist preacher.

The gullibility of royalty in the choice of medical advisers seems quite remarkable in the light of the progress then being made in anatomy and physiology. It was surpassed only by the gullibility of Parliament itself a few years later when a woman quack, Joanna Stephens, had the effrontery to announce that she would disclose her "secret cure" for the stone for the sum of £5,000. The subscription list that was opened, headed by the Duke of Richmond and two bishops, reached only £2,000. Incredible as it may seem, in 1738 Parliament voted that the balance of £3,000 be paid from public funds! In the event Joanna's "secret remedy" proved to consist of such well-tried ingredients as calcined egg shells, snails, carrot seeds and hips-and-haws, together with soap and honey, surely one of the most costly prescriptions of all time. But Joanna collected her money and, like the wise woman she was, quietly vanished from the scene.

Joanna was by no means the only person to collect a large sum of money for a cure, though she may well have been the first quack to do so. Nearly a century before, Dr. Goddard, a well-known and respectable physician and Fellow of the Royal Society, had sold the formula of his famous Goddard's Drops to Charles II for £6,000. The Drops were supposed to be a cure for everything and consisted of aromatic spirits of ammonia in solution, the active ingredient of smelling-salts. This demonstrates the very thin borderline between quackery and legitimate medicine. A quack might sell a product which actually did some good, while a qualified physician sold a cure under his own name of only doubtful value. Which, then, was the quack? The public certainly paid good money to both. If royalty and even the Government were willing to pay large sums to acquire these secret remedies, one could hardly blame the public for assuming that what they had to offer was of value.

From very early times much importance has been placed on the diagnosis of disease by the examination of urine. The eighteenth-century quack did not overlook this vital fluid, available from most patients in reasonable quantities. There were many specialists in this field, who claimed to diagnose disease merely by examining the urine and often without ever seeing the patient. These "piss-prophets" charged only a small fee for the so-called analysis of the urine, yet demanded a high price for the medicine required to cure the condition. An eighteenth century volume on *Medical Impostors* warns against them in no uncertain terms :

"Whoever hangs out a piss-pot for his standard, pretends upon sight of your water to tell your infirmities and directs medicine without seeing the sick person, believe them not. They are cheats : not only for the sixpence or shilling for what they call casting your urine (which much better would be cast in their faces), but for drawing you in with some fearful story of your danger and make you take a packet with you of their stuff."

Opponents of the piss-prophets found it easy to prove the falsity of their claims. A well-known German quack called Meyerbach was sent a flask of cow's urine for analysis purporting to have come from a middle-aged man. He diagnosed "too great great a pleasure in women." Urine analysis still remains slightly suspect in the popular view and endless stories abound supposedly demonstrating its failures. A modern version tells of the farmer who, by mistake, sent a bottle of a well-known brand of beer to his vet instead of a sample of

Doctor FREDERICK,
Lately come from *Germany*.

BEGS leave to acquaint the Publick, that he undertakes to Cure the Gout, and Rheumatifm, without any return ; being the firft perfon that ever could Cure the Gout in *London* ; Likewife, Cures the yellow Jaundice, Stitching in the Side. He likewife Cures any Body who is bit by a Mad Dog : Gentlemen and Ladies, I call myfelf Mafter; in a Word if you will make Trial where the Public may find great Benefit. No Cure no Pay.

Direct to me at Mr. *Compton's*, the *Crown* and *Feathers*; in *Holbourn*, near *Red Lyon Street*, LONDON.

9 "No cure, no pay"—a medical advertisement

animal urine. The report came back, "This horse is unfit for work and should be slaughtered immediately."

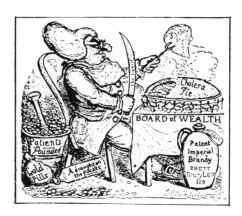

10 The rich doctor, cartoon by George Cruikshank

The procession of quacks to England from the Continent was not a one-way process; many Englishmen went abroad where they could often obtain medical qualifications with greater ease than at home. One such was John Taylor, an apothecary's assistant from Norwich, who travelled widely in Europe and in the process collected medical degrees from the universities of Basle, Liège and Cologne. When he returned to England in 1736 he was made Royal Oculist to George II.

The Hanoverians seem to have been easily impressed by a veneer of medical knowledge for a contemporary of Taylor, the famous Joshua Ward, received royal patronage and made a fortune as a result. So highly did Ward think of himself that in his will he directed that he should be buried in Westminster Abbey "within the altar rails or as near to them as possible." The Dean and Chapter thought otherwise, and Ward is buried elsewhere, but his statue still dominates the entrance to the building of the Royal Society in London.

Several quacks had begun their careers as assistants to apothecaries, as Taylor had done. Perhaps more of a charlatan than a quack was John Tawell, also from Norfolk, who, in 1810, came to London as one of the first commercial travellers in the wholesale drug trade.

Convicted of forgery, he was transported to Botany Bay in 1812, but once on parole he used his pharmaceutical knowledge and business acumen to establish the first and eventually the largest drug store in Sydney. Most of his money came from property deals, though on his premises he had consulting rooms where he advised on the popular topic of "early excesses." As a confirmed womanizer he may well have been in a position to do this, though in Australia he claimed to be a Quaker and habitually dressed as such. He even built the massive Quaker meeting-house in McQuarrie Street, Sydney, and presented it to the Society of Friends. This fact caused members much embarrassment when later he returned to England, murdered his ex-mistress with prussic acid in Slough, and was hanged outside the County Hall at Aylesbury in 1845.

The biggest quack fortunes were made in America, mainly from the treatment of supposed sexual disorders, during the nineteenth century. This was usually done by means of "Medical Institutes" with museums attached to which the public was invited free. Inside were displayed several waxwork representations, all highly coloured, purporting to show the effect of venereal disease, "self-abuse" and loose living. Syphilitic sores complete in every detail competed for attention with drooling figures alleged to be the result of masturbation, the combined effect being so repulsive and nauseating that the casual visitor could scarcely avoid feeling ill at the sight. And this was exactly what was intended. "Floormen" were constantly in attendance, and at the first sign of a queasy customer would come forward to offer sympathy and advice. A few questions were asked about the victim's general state of health, and he was very quickly persuaded that he was showing the first signs of v.d. and should immediately have a free consultation with the "specialist" upstairs. Once in the spider's web it was only a matter of minutes before the diagnosis was confirmed, but hope was held out that if the victim embarked on a course of treatment (with an immediate cash deposit) the "rummy" could be saved from an early grave.

In his *Natural History of Quackery* Eric Jameson describes these places in detail and comments on the care with which the floormen were chosen for their task. Usually they were well-educated young men who could talk convincingly, but who had temporarily fallen

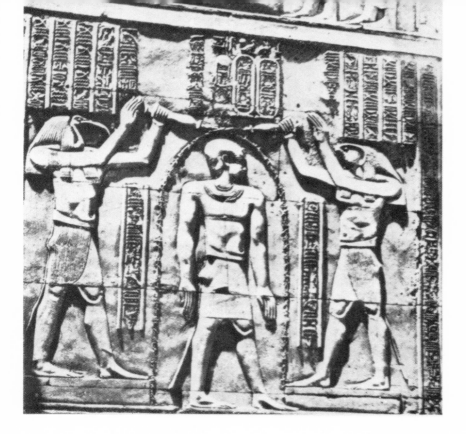

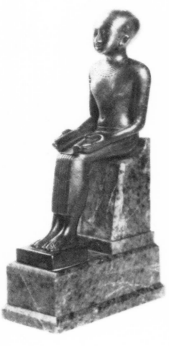

1 *Above* Pouring the
water of life over
the King, a
carving on the
walls of the
temple of
Komombo.
2 *Left* Imhotep, the
Egyptian God of
the physicians.

3. *Below* Medieval physicians treating a royal personage.

4 *Top right* Henry IV of France touching for the King's Evil.

5 *Bottom right* A knight cures a king by applying the Holy Grail to his wound, from a 14th-century French illustration from the *Roman de Lancelot*.

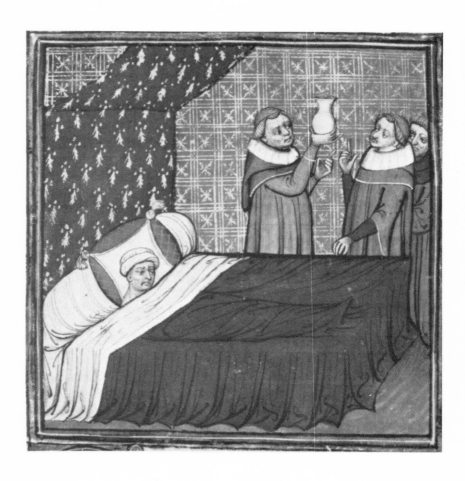

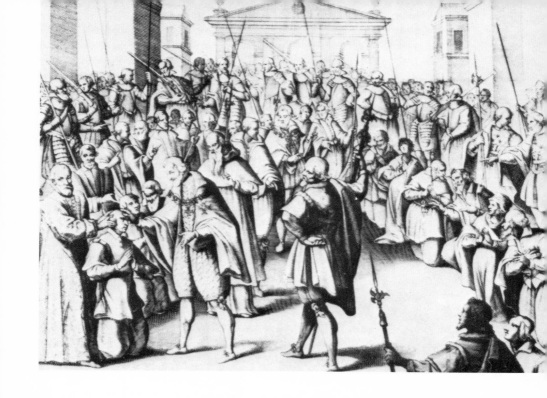

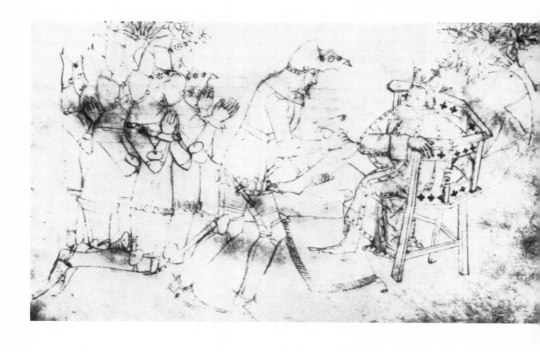

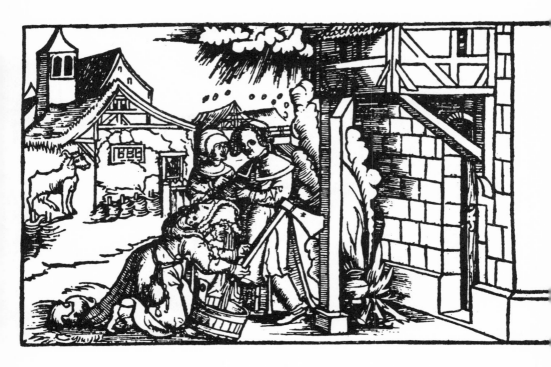

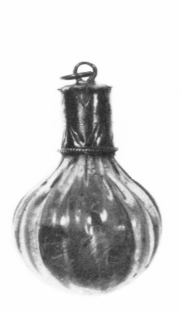
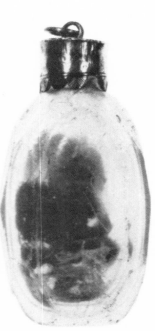

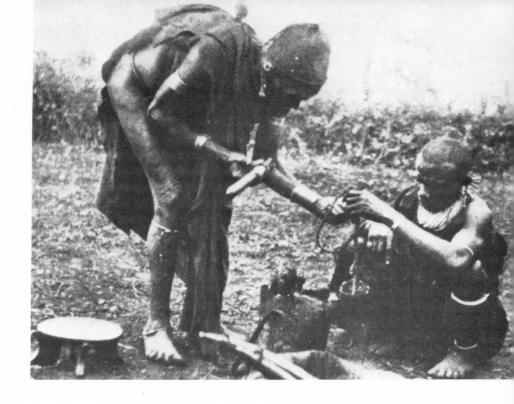

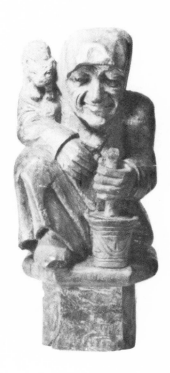

6 *Top left* A witch drawing milk from the handle of an axe, from a German woodcut of 1517.

7 & 8 *Bottom left* Bottles containing thread and mounted with silver, used to ward off the Evil Eye, from Sicily.

9 *Top right* A medicine man making a charm for protection against lions in Africa.

10 *Bottom right* An amulet in the figure of a witch with a cat on her shoulder, from France.

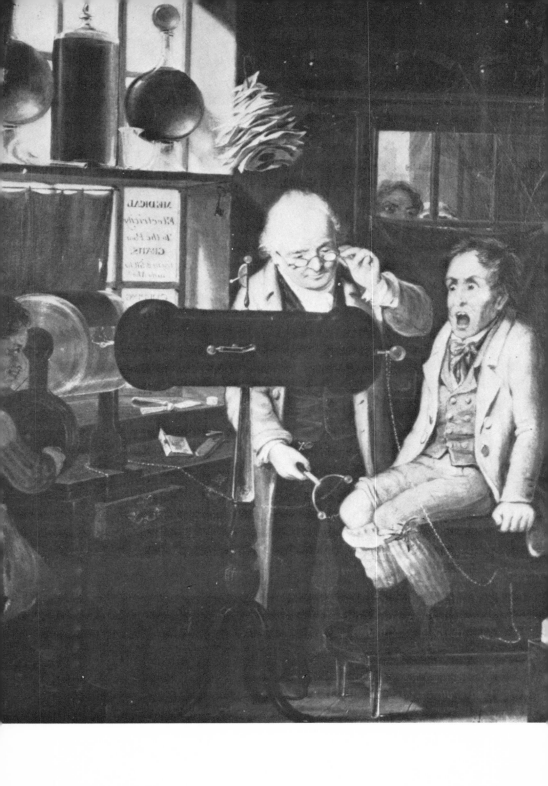

11 *Left* A satirical painting of medical electricity by Edmond Bristow (1787–1876).

12 *Top right* A caricature of 1825 of the interior of a chemist's shop with a hypochondriac on the left and an apprentice on the right.

13 *Below* "Comforts of Bath", Thomas Rowlandson's drawing of taking the waters in the time of Beau Nash.

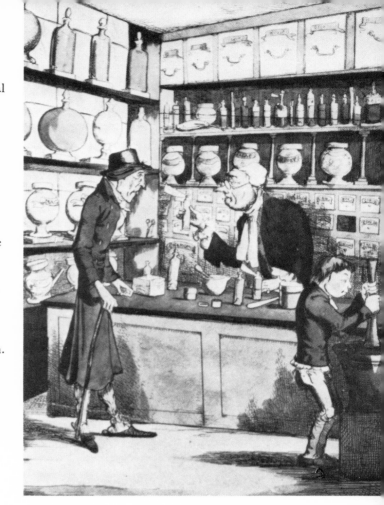

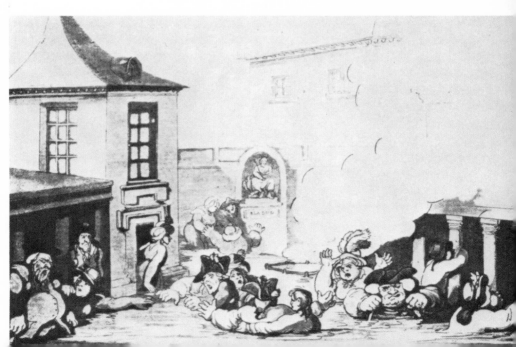

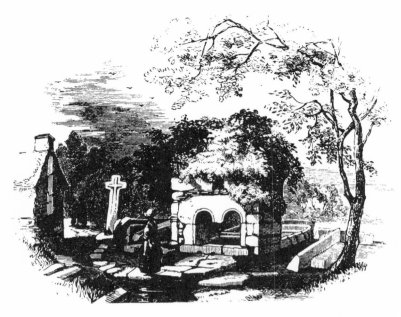

14 *Top* St. Clare's well at Liskeard in Cornwall, famous for its supposed power of curing mental disorders.

15 *Bottom* A prehistoric crickstone near Lanyon Quoist – "Go through the stone without touching it and you will never have rheumatism."

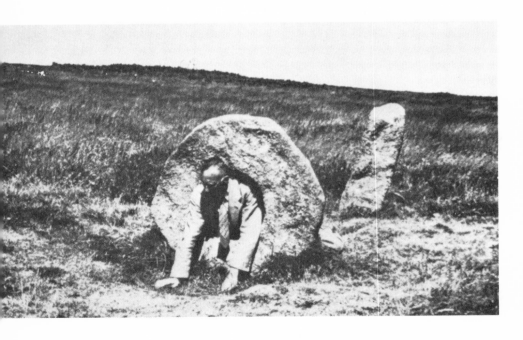

on hard times and seized the chance of earning good money, for the job was very well paid. By the turn of the century in America such establishments were causing a public scandal, and the press was taking an interest in their activities. Reporters, previously certified in good health by legitimate doctors, went to the Institutes, and were predictably informed that their days were numbered unless they took an expensive course of treatment. One of the worst cases concerned the Detroit Institute of Kennedy and Kennedy. A young immigrant was informed by this organization that he had only a few weeks to live, but could be saved by immediate treatment which involved the down payment of 150 dollars. The young man, who was about to get married, was greatly distressed by this news but did not have this sum with him. He went home to fetch the money, but instead of returning to the institute, bought a revolver and shot himself. The subsequent post-mortem showed that, in fact, he was in perfect health, and the Kennedy "specialist" spent the next few months in the State penitentiary. The directors fled the country and all over America dozens of such institutes hurriedly closed their doors.

Almost as popular with the quacks as the curing of sexual disorders was the promise to treat habitual drunkenness. The most famous quack in this field by far was Dr. Lesley Keeley, a qualified physician once employed on the medical staff of the Chicago and Alton Railroad Company. Once again it is difficult to decide whether Keeley was a quack or not. His treatment was based on injecting gold bichloride, a substance never proved to have any therapeutic properties of this nature, and of which little was known. Yet drunks from all over the United States beat a zigzag path to the doors of the Keeley Institute at Dwight, Illinois, or were lifted off trains at the impressive granite station, and given an immediate injection on the platform after they had signed the necessary contract. There is evidence that the "cure" often succeeded, though perhaps not 90 per cent as claimed by Keeley. Any success is more likely to have been due, not to the gold injections —which were stopped after the first few days—but to the patient's gradual weaning from alcohol. An important part of the regimen was that no patient should be refused alcohol, but that it should be provided in ever-decreasing amounts until the desire had gone. This technique is still in use today. The follow-on medicine consisted mainly of a concoction of cheap sherry, and it is notable how many nineteenth-century cures for alcoholism in fact consisted of mixtures of quite high alcoholic content.

At the peak of his career Keeley had Institutes in about forty cities in America including Texas, Kansas, and Philadelphia. He also tried to form a chain in England, but he met opposition from the British Medical Association and other professional bodies and the British Keeley Institute never came into being, mainly as the result of a report written about it by an Australian doctor in the most scathing terms. But Keeley may have been on the right lines. He died in 1900 after amassing a fortune, and the Keeley Institute still exists today. It is now under new management and treats alcoholism by psychiatry and orthodox medical methods. Gold bichloride is noticeably absent in the cure.

Another highly profitable venture during the nineteenth century, both in Britain and America, was in the sale of various electrical appliances for health. Dr. Graham's "Electro-Magnetico" bed was only the forerunner of hundreds of such appliances bought with gusto by the Victorian public. In London the Medical Battery Company of Oxford Street did big business with several contraptions designed for use in the home. They included the Patent Electrical Eye Battery, a normal eye-bath in which was a small battery. Diligent application to the eye thrice daily was said to cure "specks before the eyes and weakness of vision resulting from advancing age or early excesses." From the same firm came the Electropathic Belt (not to be confused with an earlier reference to electrical phenomena during sexual activity!) said to give vitality to the internal organs, to "relax morbid contractions and RENEW NERVE FORCE."

The Anti-Rheumatic Electric Towel Company of Manchester sold the Electric Towel to sufferers from neuralgia, constipation and liver disorders, advising that the product could be obtained from all chemists and "respectable drapers." Presumably they had a secret list of disreputable drapers who were refused supplies. Dr. Scott's Electric Hairbrush not only cured dandruff but also "soothed the weary brain"—and there were many others.

Most curious of all were the mechanical devices designed to provide home exercise and stimulus for those who led sedentary lives.

By far the best-known were the products of the aptly-named Vigor Company of Baker Street, London. In 1895 they were doing enormously well with their Horse-Action Saddle, a massive piece of equipment resembling a concertina mounted on a rigid iron frame, the whole topped by a full-size riding saddle with handlebars. Seated upon the saddle the rider could adjust the machine to "trot, canter or gallop." At least there was nothing to sweep up except the occasional nut and bolt.

According to the ads the Horse-Action Saddle was popular with the nobility and aristocracy, a curious claim since most such people might be expected to have their own horses. Nevertheless, no less than the Princess Alexandra of Wales had "personally" ordered one, no doubt to pass the time away during Prince Edward's protracted absences from home. What Alexandra thought of the machine is unrecorded. But there is no doubt what the Countess of Aberdeen felt about it. "The Horse-Saddle," she declared in her testimonial, "has given me complete satisfaction."

In New England in the 1790s a country doctor named Elisha Perkins began to advertise his Metallic Tractors. His idea, and one that was already the basis of almost world-wide superstition, was that disease could be drawn out of the body by some metal object. Perkins Tractors consisted of a pair of four-inch rods of metal tapered at one end. With the blunt ends held together the pointed ends were placed on the body and drawn downward and outward in a gentle stroking movement. Perkins' own claims were initially modest enough. He maintained they would cure headache, stomach-ache backache and rheumatism, though later he added to the list paralysis and "minor deformities." Much to the doctor's own surprise the most fantastic successes were soon being announced by those who had tried Tractoration, as the treatment came to be called. Testimonials poured in from many well-known and famous people, and George Washington himself is said to have used the Tractors. Perkins jumped on the bandwagon, taking more and more space in the newspapers to advertise his product and pushing the price up to $25 a pair. The craze had gained a firm grip, and even censure from the Connecticut Medical Associations and Perkins' removal from the register failed to stem the tide. When a Danish diplomat returned home he took a pair of Tractors with him, and within months Tractoration had begun to sweep through Europe. Perkins died in 1799 of Yellow Fever after travelling to New York to launch his latest product—a cure for Yellow Fever! His son carried on the good work and visited Britain to introduce the Tractors to an eager public. He had premises in the West End of London and, once again, the nobility beat a path to his door. It is curious that in this instance, unlike that of Keeley and his gold injections a century later, the English medical profession approved of the treatment while the American certainly did not. They approved so enthusiastically that in 1803 a Perkineaean Institute was actually opened in Soho in London where the poor who could not afford Tractors of their own were treated free. This was probably Perkins' undoing, for immediately complaints began coming in that the treatment was no good. As every confidence trickster knows, people who have been duped rarely complain to the authorities. But the National Health Service has also proved that nobody complains more loudly about medical treatment than those who are getting it free.

By 1810 the bubble had burst. Perkins returned to America some £10,000 richer than when he had arrived in England, and the "drawing-out" of disease with metal returned to the province of folk-medicine where it remains today. Other cults were to follow later, creating fortunes for their practitioners. In 1895 Hercules Sanche in America was doing well with his Electropoise, a short length of metal gas-pipe attached to the body by an adjustable strap. It was said to supply "the needed amount of electrical force to the system and place the body in condition to absorb the oxygen through lungs and pores." An improved version of the Electropoise was Sanche's Oxydonor where the instrument was attached to the wrist or ankle and a metal lead provided which was placed in a bowl of water. The patient then settled down to thumb his way through the pages of the latest issue of the *Journal of the American Medical Association* while the Oxydonor did its healthful work. There was even a special attachment for married couples by which the appliance could be attached to both pairs of ankles in bed, the lead then running to a filled receptacle conveniently placed underneath! Sanche was one of the first to see the advantages of optional extras for his gadgets, and also to invent a Users' Club, which he called the Fraternity of Duxanimae. Incredibly, it was still alive in 1950.

In England Dr. Mattei's "Electrical Fluid" was enjoying good sales at the turn of the century until analysed by the British Medical Association, who proved it to be nothing but tap-water. It killed the product, though others of only doubtful value survived such poor publicity. Notable was Lydia Pinkham's Vegetable Compound, in America, and Mother Seigel's Syrup in England, both of which made fortunes for their proprietors.

An ingenious quack at the beginning of the nineteenth century was the engaging Irishman John St. John Long, who worked in London in the 1820s. Long specialized in tuberculosis, a good choice in an age when "consumption" claimed so many young lives. He supplied an ointment which had to be rubbed on all parts of the body and any sign of irritation or discolouration of the skin was supposed to prove that the ointment was "extracting" the disease. Yet there were also the inherent risks that consumption would prove fatal, and there is evidence that Long purposely chose from his patients many who were not suffering from the disease, to demonstrate a "cure" later on. Surprisingly, he survived two trials for manslaughter when patients died after treatment; he was fined £250 on one charge but acquitted on the other. So great was public confidence in him that the second victim was actually the wife of a man who had seen him convicted at his first trial! Long was a very handsome young man and loved by women. He was careful that no breath of scandal should ever touch him, was particularly careful in his dealings with women patients. He never married, though no doubt had many opportunities. After a brief excursion into treating mental illness by "extracting fluid from the brain" he finally succumbed from the disease he had claimed to cure and died of tuberculosis in 1834. He left the secret of his ointment to his brother, saying that the formula was worth £10,000 on the open market. Unfortunately there were no buyers.

Even if the treatment and products sold by some quacks were virtually useless they sowed the seeds of ideas that have blossomed into this century and become respectable. A classic example is the science of osteopathy evolved by the American Civil War officer

Andrew Taylor Still. He maintained that "there are no such diseases as Fever, Typhus, Rheumatism, Gout, Colic, Liver diseases or Croup." All human ills could be cured by correct manipulation of the spine. "God is the Father of Osteopathy," he proudly announced. "And I am not ashamed of the child of His mind." It has since been proved that incorrect bone-positioning can cause many functional disorders and in the 1930s the famous English osteopath, Sir Herbert Barker, showed how much the medical profession still had to learn about bone manipulation.

Very different were the many remedies for bad and aching teeth that have contributed nothing to modern dental techniques. St. Apollonia was the patron saint of dentistry, and samples of her teeth were widely sold in fifteenth-century England as a cure for toothache. Unfortunately the number of holy teeth on the market far exceeded the capabilities of even a saint, and Edward VI banned the sale of the teeth and ordered all stocks to be confiscated. According to Dr. John Fuller "a veritable ton of teeth was thus collected."

Bones, too, have always been popular when infants are teething, and bones thought to be those of a saint were particularly valued. The bones of St. Hugh were highly prized. This man was extremely fond of children and was said to comfort them by stroking their gums after he had dipped his fingers in holy water. No doubt St. Hugh was as well set up with bones as St. Apollonia was with teeth, though there is no record of any collection of these items being made.

Though not as numerous as quack doctors, quack dentists were plentiful in the eighteenth century and were a popular attraction at fairs and markets in Europe and America. One of the most famous was Martin van Butchall who was one of the sights of London in the 1770s. He claimed to be able to supply a complete set of dentures and fit them "without drawing stumps or causing pain." If true, this would have made him famous enough without the additional publicity he created by riding round London on a white horse painted with purple spots. As an additional and slightly macabre advertisement he also kept in his permanent London home the embalmed body of his dead wife. She was dressed in a fine lace gown, with carmine injected into her veins, and matching glass eyes. Butchall's second wife objected to this constant reminder of her predecessor, and the dentist presented the mummy to the Royal College of Surgeons where it remained on display until destroyed by a German bomb in 1941.

A century before van Butchall, David Perronet was selling his tooth-paste, guaranteed to make "black teeth as ivory," and in Paris Le Grand Thomas, an enormous man said to sleep eighteen hours a day, sold a specific which "cured radically every secret disease" and

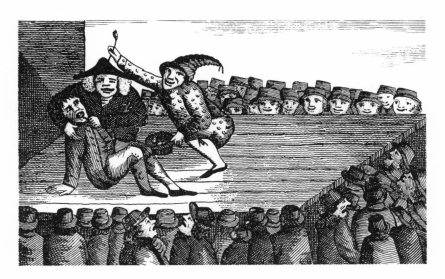

11 A quack dentist performing on stage

also extracted teeth "without pain but not without the unfolding of great strength."

An example of a British quack product attributed to American folk medicine was Sequar's Oil and Prairie Flower Mixture, two toothache cures on sale in London before World War One. They were said to have been invented by the Sioux and Cherokee Indians. Unfortunately for the makers, a government analyst showed the Oil was merely turpentine and fish oil, and the Prairie Flowers bicarbonate of soda and aloes.

Aloes was a favourite ingredient of many quack remedies, and was the "prime mover" of that famous medicine of its day, Morison's Universal Vegetable Compound. This medicine, like Beecham's Pills fifty years later, depended on its purgative qualities for its success. And James Morison certainly found success when he brought his remedy to London and began business in 1805 during the Regency period. Morison also took advantage of the uninhibited times in which he lived and warmly recommended flagellation as a cure for illness. This was, in any case, a popular pastime and several establishments were run for this purpose presided over by ladies known as "whippers". One of the best known in Regency London was Mrs. Berkeley, who owned premises near Portland Place. She invented the famous "Berkeley Horse," a curious kind of padded trestle upon which customers could be whipped to their hearts' content. Morison got a percentage from these good ladies for any customers ready to convince themselves they were taking Morison's medical treatment instead of merely finding a new way to arouse their jaded sexual appetites.

Morison was one of the few quacks who seemed to believe in his own medicine. He took his Vegetable Compound all his life, died at the age of seventy and left £500,000. He was buried with much pomp in Kensal Green in a tomb almost the size of a house.

8

Faith and Healing

THE idea that illness and disease were brought about by the displeasure of the gods has meant that the art of healing has always been closely linked with religious beliefs. Such beliefs did not always help medical progress, for as religious thought became more organized, and a single God displaced the many gods of ancient times, the rights and wrongs of man-made healing became a major issue.

Some people felt that illness should be cured by the wonders of Nature that God himself had provided. Others, including the early Christian Church, held that any attempts to heal the sick were sinful in that they sought to circumvent the wishes of the Almighty. A third view, which gained more adherents as time went on, especially the Roman Catholic Church, was that with faith miraculous cures could be brought about by God's direct intervention through the saints. Today this is seen in the annual pilgrimage to Lourdes and Lisieux, and in medieval England resulted in the famous pilgrimages to places such as Walsingham, to the shrine of Thomas à Becket in Canterbury and to the holy well of Blessed John Schorne in North Marston, Buckinghamshire.

This is a very different kind of faith from the mysticism found in eastern countries, where intense and absolute concentration over long periods can even result in the body no longer being able to feel pain. The Indian yogi walking barefoot over red hot coals is one example; another are the priests in Nigeria who allow their tongues to be transfixed with a metal spike apparently without pain. The Yoga Research Centre at Hyderabad has recently conducted tests on such phenomena as live burial, and has shown that during a trance the metabolism of the body virtually stops. Temperature falls, breathing almost ceases, and the pulse is almost imperceptible. Experienced yogi rarely suffer from illness and maintain a youthful vigour well into old age. The work of the Centre may eventually benefit science and reveal some of the secrets of the ageing process.

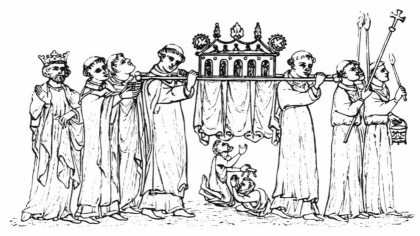

12 Miraculous cures from relics

In the west yoga has only recently begun to attract interest. It is used mainly in the form of short periods of concentration and exercise designed to maintain good health. However, many students, especially from America, are visiting India to study the cult at close range. It may provide a sympathetic ambience for those who consider that worldly problems are best solved by withdrawing from them. Yoga has been practised in India for many centuries, but the rigid caste system and mass poverty does not inspire confidence in any social benefits from yoga. Yet India does have one community which seems to have found the secret of long life and happiness. This is the independent monarchy of Hunza, whose people are said to be originally of Caucasian stock. For two thousand years they have lived in a remote and inaccessible region high in the Himalayas of north-west India. Here, protected from the outside world by the soaring white peaks, they pursue an existence that may well have been the model for James Hilton's Shangri-La. There are no police, jails or army, no juvenile delinquency and the last reported misdemeanour by an adult was in 1830! The few scientists and doctors who have visited this region have reported an environment so apparently perfect and idyllic that one would scarcely believe it existed had not their findings been reported in the serious journals.

From these reports it appears that most of the people live to be a hundred or more, retaining perfect physical and mental fitness to the end. Sickness is virtually non-existent and the modern scourges of cancer, high blood-pressure, stomach ulcers and heart disease are unknown. Even the children do not suffer from the ailments we all expect in the western world.

The secret of the Hunza people and their near-perfect existence rests on three things: Firstly their determination not to be contaminated by modern influences; secondly the particular type of yoga which is a basic part of their religion; and thirdly the diet by which they live. Yoga allows them complete powers of relaxation, and in their daily work they will often pause, allow the body to relax, and remain in a trance for several minutes before resuming their toil. They take the view that life is divided into three parts—the young years, the middle years, and the rich years. This is a very different attitude of mind from that of our so-called civilized communities, where too much importance may often be attached to the affairs of the young and too little to the needs and welfare of the old.

Again, Hunza people never retire from work, in the western sense, believing that the idleness of retirement is a far greater enemy to life than work. They are careful to work slowly, remaining cheerful at all times and have never developed the acquisitive and competitive attitude of other societies. Their small administrative system is mainly devoted to keeping outsiders at bay. Quite apart from the terrifying ordeal of the journey (which can be made only at certain times of the year) travellers may visit Hunza only by direct invitation from the King himself and on a special permit issued personally by the President of Pakistan.

As to their diet, Hunza people eat mainly cereals and wholemeal bread, green vegetables, potatoes, milk, cheese butter and fruit. Eggs are scarce and have only recently been imported. They rarely eat meat, but drink a highly potent wine made from grapes. Most of the food is eaten raw. The benefits of this way of life seem to be that men of eighty have the physique of westeners half that age, and happily continue to father children until well into their nineties. Their faith in life is simple and strong, but above all they have learned the power of relaxation.

More common than yoga in Europe and America is the belief that bodily illnesses can be cured through spiritualism, with a medium acting as intermediary between the living and the spirits of the departed. A different kind of faith again is found in the beliefs of the Christian Scientists who maintain that bodily illness does not exist at all, but is purely an illusion. This is the fundamental difference between Christian Science and other similar religions, for even though the symptoms of disease are held to be only "in the mind," this is not considered to be the result of any psychiatric disturbance. According to the Christian Scientists illnesses simply do not exist, and to them psychiatric treatment is as useless and mischievous as recourse to medicine. This is the theory. In practice things are rather different. Concessions have been made since the movement was first launched by Mary Baker Eddy in America in 1877. Vaccination is permitted and also medical attention at childbirth and when in pain. This is explained by saying that ordinary men and women do not have enough will-power to rid themselves of what they *think* they are suffering from. Opiates and drugs may be allowed to help the Christian Scientist rid himself of the belief that he is actually ill. Christian Science found many devotees during the life of its founder, and on her death in 1910 there were nearly seven hundred churches in the United States alone. Half a century later it is a world-wide organization with some three thousand churches.

Christian Scientists apart, most cultures, both primitive and sophisticated, take the view that sickness and disease exist and can be cured by appeals to God, Nature, the Spirit World, or some other higher authority. Even so, this conviction can be selective, and not all illnesses are accepted as such. In certain African tribes the prevalence of yaws—a contagious disease akin to leprosy—is so high that those who do not contract it are considered abnormal and viewed with suspicion. North Amazonian Indians who do not exhibit the disfiguring symptoms of endemic syphilis are thought to lack virility and find it hard to marry.

Where the presence of disease is accepted by primitive tribes, the

108

method of cure, as we have seen, is usually a mixture of faith, magic, and medicine. But in ancient civilized cultures the sudden onset of disease as a mark of divine displeasure might have to be stemmed by direct appeal to the gods through atonement or sacrifice; no normal therapeutic measures would be enough. The Old Testament tells how the Philistines defeated the Jews at Ebenezer, stealing the Ark of the Covenant and carrying it off to Ashdod. As a result the Philistines were visited with bubonic plague of such severity that the priests and diviners were forced to advise the immediate return of the Ark to the Jews together with "guilt" offerings of gold.

An interesting aspect of this story is that the gift was ordered to be in the form of golden rats, an animal now known to be a carrier of bubonic plague. Though this is unlikely to have been known at the time, the death of many rats as a precursor to an epidemic seems to have been noticed by the ancients. In the cruel religion of the Mexican Aztecs the priests habitually cut open the chests of living men and tore out their hearts, offering them to the sun god as a sacrifice and propitiation at times of plague or pestilence.

The connection between sin and disease has persisted in the human mind well into modern times and within civilized communities. It has often helped to prolong disease and acted as a barrier to its cure. In 1832, when cholera first reached the United States from Europe via Canada, New York preachers thundered against the sins of gluttony, drink and sexual excess prevalent in the slum areas where the cholera first struck, and pronounced it as "God's justice" against the sinners. The Catholic Bishop of Philadelphia preached that cholera was a visitation of God, and the *Western Sunday School Messenger* treated its youthful readers to the following: "Drunkards and filthy, wicked people of all descriptions, are swept away in heaps, as if the Holy God could no longer bear their wickedness, just as we sweep away a mass of filth when it has become so corrupt that we cannot bear it. The cholera is not *caused* by intemperance and filth in themselves, but it is a *scourge*, a *rod*, in the hand of God."

Almost every sect united to condemn the cholera's first victims, most of them illiterate Irish Catholic immigrants. Not until after the second outbreak in 1849 did the view of cholera as "the scourge of the sinful" begin to decline, partly as people realized that it also struck down the honest and the upright and partly through a new awareness of the shocking and insanitary conditions that bred the disease. Even so, a leader in the *Ohio Observer* stated that the end of the epidemic was "striking proof, to the nation and to the world, that we are a religious and Christian nation."

Christian and religious the nation may have been, but it was certainly not united in its religious beliefs. Religious sects began to proliferate in America in the early nineteenth century when conventional religion was felt by many to be inadequate. The New World saw the founding of all kinds of creeds—the Mormons, Seventh Day Adventists, Christian Scientists and Christadelphians. It also adopted many strange religious cults from Europe including the Amish sect from Germany and the Dukhobors from Russia. In the Southern States slaves from Africa had imported their own brands of witchcraft and superstition, later to be grafted on to Christian creeds. Britain, too, was showing more diversity. Not for nothing did a nineteenth-century French traveller remark in despair that "England has two hundred religions, but only one soup."

Most sects had moderate views on matters of health and sickness. These included the Mormons who today, with an estimated world membership of $2\frac{1}{2}$ million, can claim to be one of the most successful of latter-day religions. Their beliefs in how to preserve good health are reasonable and include abstention from tobacco, alcohol, hot drinks such as tea, cocoa and coffee, "and all other drugs and narcotics." In this they hold similar views to the Seventh Day Adventists, founded by William Miller in New York State in 1834. When his prophecies about the end of the world failed to materialize Miller withdrew from the scene, but his place was taken by a disciple, the extraordinary seventeen-year-old epileptic, Ellen G. Harmon, better known after her third marriage as Ellen G. White. Ellen had visions all her life until her death in 1915. According to witnesses, she seemed to enter a trance during these visions, during which her breathing stopped completely —a fact vouched for by various "physicians of skill." Her muscles remained fixed and rigid though she could move her arms, and in fact could hold for thirty minutes in one frail hand an eighteen-pound bible that she could not lift with both hands in her normal state. She was also gifted with the power of healing and there are several accounts of her "miraculous" cures. Ellen's vast output of writings during a long life includes many instructions on diet as the way to preserve health. The drinking of hot beverages was forbidden as they "excited the baser passions and created unnatural appetites." Meat was forbidden, and pork in particular, in her view, was responsible for scrofula, leprosy and cancer. Sugar was a sure source of disease, and cakes and custards made from sugar, milk and eggs were particularly harmful. Little was left on the menu, but this did not matter, for Sister White maintained that the first lesson of all was to deny the appetite. It was sinful to "cultivate taste."

Modern Seventh Day Adventists still follow these strict dietary rules based on the "unclean meats" listed in the Book of Leviticus. The sect is undoubtedly rigid and authoritarian, yet turns its precepts into good account and as a source of income by manufacturing and selling various breads and cereal products under the brand-name Granose. It is also the only religious sect with its own medical school whose degrees are accepted by the medical profession. Its qualified physicians spread the gospel of diet and health throughout the world.

The creed of another highly successful sect, Jehovah's Witnesses, includes amongst its many tenets at least one which is medically important. Based on an interpretation of various Old Testament texts their refusal to accept blood transfusions often results in wide publicity, particularly if a Witness dies as a result. The most important text invoked is "Ye shall eat the blood of no manner of flesh" which, for Witnesses, includes the assimilation of blood into the body in any manner. Many have died through clinging tenaciously to this doctrine. Far more numerous are those who have died as a result of another principle of their creed—refusal to undertake military service. During World War Two more than six thousand Witnesses died in German concentration camps and nearly four thousand went to prison in America. In Canada and Australia the sect was declared illegal for the duration of the war but in Britain, though suspected of trying to influence soldiers to desert by means of carefully planted girl friends, their activities were not curtailed.

In America, since the war, H. W. Armstrong and his Radio Church of God have thundered against the sins of the nation, forecasting plagues and epidemics starting in 1965 and ending in 1972, with a third of the population dead. Undaunted by the fact that this has not happened, they now confidently predict that America will soon be attacked by the "Ten-Nation European Colossus" (perhaps the Common Market?) led by a *fuehrer* even more terrible than Hitler. The attack will be by atom bomb, killing most of the population. Those remaining will expire of epidemic diseases including a plague of "boils from head to foot." The Church's magazine, *The Plain Truth*, obligingly illustrates this unpleasant condition so that the faithful will readily recognize the symptoms.

It is a relief to turn to those religions that promise relief from sickness and cures for disease as part of their creed. Not that all of them are entirely innocent. Now and again men have set themselves up as prophets of a new faith mingling religion with healing—sometimes with disastrous results. One such man was Josef Weissenberg, a seventy-year-old ex-cabby and waiter, who founded his "New Jerusalem" in Berlin in the 1920s. Had it been merely another way-out religious cult, or had Weissenberg been just another quack, little would have been heard of him. But a woman was declared insane after trying to murder her husband as a result of his administrations, and the police began to take notice. Their interest was further aroused by the discovery that members of the cult, "The Community of St. John," were not reporting the death of relatives to the authorities, but waiting patiently for the Master to bring them back to life. It also became clear that Weissenberg was treating many complaints with a curious form of therapy consisting of faith, prayer and cream cheese, the latter specially manufactured on his dairy farm outside Berlin. Weissenberg never explained this part of the treatment, except to say that he used it "under Divine guidance." When a believer who was a diabetic died after the treatment the Master was arrested and charged with criminal neglect. A second charge at the same hearing involved the tragic case of a baby girl with poor eyesight whose parents were members of the cult and who had used the cream-cheese cure. Within a few weeks the baby had been blinded for life. Astonishingly, though convicted on the second charge (the diabetic was deemed to have died of natural causes), Weissenberg successfully appealed and was released from prison. A later death saw him in court again, this time convicted and sentenced to six months' imprisonment. He died before commencing his sentence and after lodging another appeal, and his following declined. By then it was 1933, and the latest of the New Jerusalems was forgotten in the excitement surrounding an even more pernicious cult—the rise of National Socialism and the beginning of the "millennium" of German supremacy.

Weissenberg was not the only man to have founded a new religion based on the treatment of disease. More eccentric still was Johannes Binggeli, founder of the Forest Brotherhood in Switzerland in the 1890s. His religion had as its mainstay the belief that sexual intercourse was a cure for all ills—and he was its high-priest. His own genitals he described as "The Box of Christ" and his urine "heavenly balm" which his disciples eagerly used for all illnesses. Female complaints could be cured by intercourse with him, a form of therapy he practised on his own daughter and which brought him into court in 1896 when she became pregnant. Bingelli was charged with incest and convicted, but allowed to serve his sentence in a mental home instead of prison.

Men like Weissenberg and Binggeli were both religious and medical impostors. Yet in the long history of both kinds of quackery there is evidence that many people have apparently been cured, or their symptoms relieved, without any logical explanation. The knowledge that the processes of the mind are intimately associated with bodily function is nothing new. Priests in ancient Babylon made use of it when they interpreted dreams to try and diagnose illness. Today there is a mass of evidence proving that cures and healing can be brought about by other means when conventional medicine has failed. What creates dispute and argument among medical and religious thinkers is not that it happens, but exactly *how* it happens.

The most organized body claiming to heal by supranormal methods are the spiritualists. In Britain the National Federation of Spiritual Healers claims to have more than two thousand active practitioners. Since 1960, they have been given permission to attend most hospitals to treat patients. This decision caused an immediate outcry in the medical profession as it came only two years after a special B.M.A. committee of investigation had announced that "there is no evidence that there is any special type of illness cured solely by spiritual healing which cannot be cured by medical methods." The spiritualists, many doctors argued, had been allowed into hospitals on the pretext that other ministers of religion had this right, despite the fact that spiritualism and orthodox religion had little in common. The spiritualists, as a result, were careful to create an atmosphere of comfort when visiting the sick and refrained from giving any impression of mumbo-jumbo by odd behaviour such as talking with spirits or going into a trance. Under such conditions their presence was as beneficial as that of any other visitor, for the therapeutic effect of sympathy and reassurance can reduce symptoms and make the patient become less conscious of pain. There is no doubt that for many outsiders the world of spiritual healing seems to exist in a kind of vacuum suspended between orthodox religion and conventional medical practice. Both tend to be rigid in their views, the medical profession, in the past, insisting on a scientific explanation of what happens, while religious teachers hold that any "miraculous" cures must come from God and God alone. The spiritualists, convinced that the spirits of dead people can work through mediums (or "sensitives" as they prefer to be called) find opponents in both camps. Despite this, some doctors do subscribe to the beliefs of the spiritualists, as do even more churchmen. Unfortunately, little research has been done to discover just what effect a receptive state of mind has on bodily functions. The spiritualists are certain their methods work, but they make no attempt to explain the phenomenon.

A curious aspect of this kind of healing is the diversity of methods used and the differences of opinion among those who practise it. Some claim to heal across long distances, curing patients who are miles away, often in ignorance of the effort being made on their behalf and even hostile to it. This type of healing requires no faith on the part of the patient and is the reason why the term "faith-healer" is not always accepted. Others, including some clerics, take the view that disease can be cured only "when sufficient faith is present." Cures are claimed by touch, by manipulation, even by the performance of simulated operations conducted near the body and supposedly on the aura itself. The sensitive may go into a trance, or he may stay fully conscious and aware of what is happening.

Probably the actual method is unimportant. What is agreed by all such healers is that they are acting as a channel of communication between the spirit world and those still living, and that those who engaged in the art of healing when alive can still exert their influence from the other world. Harry Edwards, one of Britain's best-known spirit healers, claims to be guided by the spirits of Louis Pasteur and Lord Lister, and has an impressive clientele who share his belief. Not all spiritualists are so definite, but their followers are no less faithful. Latest estimates (1972) indicate that more than a million people every year go to spiritualists to be cured. Oddly, people will accept without question the most outrageous contentions put forward by individuals, yet there is an almost instinctive reaction to resist those propounded by responsible groups. The wish to rationalize every miracle in the Bible is almost equalled by those who insist that the results of spiritual healing could be achieved by normal medical methods. Yet the same B.M.A. committee which made that assertion in 1958 also stated that "through spiritual healing recoveries take place that cannot be explained by medical science."

Two main objections are made by doctors. (1) The patient may suffer by being diverted from accepted medical techniques. (2) Most cures are of a temporary nature and the condition often reasserts itself after a time.

As to the first objection, records show that most of those who have recourse to spiritualists do so only after undergoing orthodox medical treatment. The second objection is probably more valid, for many cures that have been followed up later show that the condition returns once the atmosphere of the healing session has waned. Many think that the fact that there has been any relief at all, however temporary, is worth attention and should be a field for much more research.

The miraculous cures claimed at Lourdes and other places of pilgrimage are far fewer, but more dramatic, than those claimed by the spiritualists. The conditions required before a cure can be considered as a miracle are so rigorous that one wonders how any have succeeded.

The criteria, imposed by the Roman Catholic Church itself, are as follows:

1.   The disease must be extremely serious and hard to cure.

2. The possibility of spontaneous remission must be eliminated.
3. Earlier medical treatment, if any, must have failed.
4. The cure must be immediate, or at least sudden.
5. The cure must be complete.
6. The cure must not be as a consequence of some natural crisis.
7. There must be no relapse.

Of the six million pilgrims who have made the journey to Lourdes since young Bernadette Soubirous saw her visions of the Virgin Mary in 1858, less than sixty people can claim to have been cured miraculously. An example of the rigid working of the tests is given by Geoffrey Murray in his *Frontiers of Healing* (1958) in describing the case of Jack Traynor. This man, wounded at Gallipoli in World War One, had been invalided out of the army with a full disability pension. Machine-gun bullets had severed the nerves of his right arm, leaving it completely paralysed. A head wound had affected the brain and made him an epileptic. He had lost all feeling in both legs and had no physical control of his bodily functions. Ten of Britain's finest surgeons had operated on him, and one such operation had left him with a hole in his skull. By all accounts Traynor was one of the worst casualties to survive that terrible war, and when he expressed his desire to travel to Lourdes his medical advisers feared for his life. He was eventually allowed to make the journey under strict medical supervision.

At Lourdes the incredible happened. Overnight his epilepsy vanished, he regained the use of his limbs and acquired control of his body, and the hole in his head disappeared! These facts were vouched for by several doctors and surgeons who had previously attended him. Nobody could explain it. Three years later Traynor was still a healthy man and expressed his intention of taking up work as a coalman! Incredible as this may seem, what seems even more extraordinary is that the Catholic Church still refuses to accept it as miracle, presumably because it does not conform to one of the above criteria. Rule 7 alone seems to debar any claim for a miraculous cure during the lifetime of the patient, for not until death can it be certain that there will be no relapse.

The Catholic Church does little to encourage a belief in miracles, for unfulfilled hopes could have tragic consequences. Lourdes developed as a place of pilgrimage during the nineteenth century despite the efforts of the Church to play down the visions of Bernadette. She herself, as a nun in later life, refused to comment on the matter. Today, when Lourdes is visited by a growing number of handicapped children, the words of the chaplain on one such pilgrimage are of interest. His instructional notes to the children includes this passage : "I expect you have heard that sometimes sick people are made better when they go to Lourdes, but you must understand that only very few are cured out of the thousands of sick persons who go. Of course, we should pray that God may make us a little better . . ." There is certainly no promise of a miracle there. Nevertheless, if only one authenticated and accepted miracle had taken place at Lourdes it would inevitably have become a place of pilgrimage. In fact, more than fifty are recorded.

Dr. William Sargant, head of the department of psychological medicine at St. Thomas's Hospital, London, is an acknowledged authority on how belief and faith can influence bodily functions, and on how physical factors can affect the mind. In an article in *World Medicine* (June, 1969) he discusses how the mind can suddenly latch on to beliefs that are apparently quite illogical and against a person's better judgement. This may be brought about by sudden changes in brain function induced by such outside stimuli as drumming and dancing, the mass emotion of a revival meeting, or by the calculated emptying of the mind as in Yoga and other forms of prolonged concentration. Either way the effect can be sudden, and in the latter process may permanently affect the subject's behavioural pattern. Under such conditions people have reported the sudden feeling of being possessed by an outside being, maybe God, Christ, the Holy Ghost, Voodoo gods, African devils or the spirit of some dead person. John Wesley himself was well aware that faith of this kind could be induced by great anxiety, guilt or mental conflict. He also knew that under these conditions a person who had previously held no firm religious convictions was highly susceptible to all similar suggestions. When preaching in Ireland, he was worried that his converts might be re-converted to the Roman Church by priests once his influence had faded.

Dr. Sargant also points out that sudden faith can be induced by methods which are the reverse of external stimuli. Abnormal brain function can be brought about by emptying the brain of all voluntary and involuntary thoughts. This may require months, even years, of practice; but the result is the same. One part of the brain concentrates on a particular object or desire to the exclusion of all extraneous matter, so that the remainder becomes virtually non-productive. A point is finally reached when the god, or whatever is the focus of concentration, is felt to enter the subject and become part of him. An example quoted is of a businessman with normally excellent judgement in everyday matters who, after some overwhelming emotional experience or after a long illness, comes to believe that all the secrets of the universe are hidden in the mathematical calculations of the pyramids. The rest of his life could well be devoted to proving his thesis, even to twisting facts to make them fit, though his judgement on all other matters remains unimpaired.

Not everyone subscribes to Dr. Sargant's view that faith is just a matter of abnormal brain function. But that brain function can be altered by the action of certain drugs is now freely accepted. The present interest in what are termed hallucinatory drugs as a short cut to religious salvation is an alarming symptom of this, though it is by no means new. Mescaline has long been used by Mexican Indians in the form of the peyote plant as part of their religious ritual. As Huxley and others discovered, mescaline appears to reveal the personal presence and certainty of God. The result of this is that while hallucinatory drugs are banned in most countries in the west, the government of Mexico has had to allow the use of the peyote plant to continue amongst Indians as being part of their religious belief.

The use of drugs to heighten perception and increase faith can result in eventual damage to the brain. In December, 1971, the British medical journal, *Lancet*, said: "Personality changes and mental illness have been reported on chronic cannabis smokers of previously normal personality. Addicts often have impairment of recent memory . . . and a tendency to reversed sleep pattern suggesting organic brain damage." Evidence of actual brain shrinkage was proved in ten young men who had been smoking cannabis for some years. The cavities, or ventricles, of the brain, enlarge, and a similar shrinkage of the surrounding tissue is found in chronic alcoholism and in some forms of epilepsy. Tests on monkeys show that cannabis is deposited in the ventricles and has the same effect. Yet such is the unwillingness of many young people to accept these findings, though carried out under strict conditions by experienced researchers, that in a recent survey* 92 per cent of California medical students and 88 per cent of Ontario medical students did not believe that physical health would be seriously impaired by cannabis. In view of the added findings that only 11 per cent of the Californian medical students would warn a cannabis-smoking patient that he was in any danger, the outlook for the future seems grim. It is, perhaps, some consolation to remember that those students who talk loudest and indulge in the most bizarre behaviour at medical school often develop into staid and highly conservative physicians later in life, and are horrified when reminded of their youthful views. Even so, outstanding talents in the arts have frequently been associated with chronic drug addiction, though harmful effects have not always followed. Samuel Taylor Coleridge (1772–1834) was boasting at the age of nineteen that opium had no ill-effect on him, and Thomas De Quincey (1785–1859), the best-known addict of all, was certain it increased his imaginative powers. He was seventy-nine when he died. On the other hand, Francis Thompson (1859–1907) wrote much poetry of a high order but succumbed to the effects of opium and other drugs at the age of forty-seven. Baudelaire became addicted to hashish at twenty and was dead at forty-five. The author Guy de Maupassant died at forty-two, twelve years after developing the habit of sniffing ether. The distorted faces and elongated necks in the paintings of Modigliani, who died at thirty-six, have been attributed by some to his addiction to hashish, which he bought as a paste and spread on bread-and-butter! A notable exception was Jean Cocteau, whose fame rests on films as much as on his literary output. A lifelong opium addict, he claimed it did him no physical harm, though admitting that it could be harmful to some. Cocteau died at seventy-four, insisting to the end that the medical profession had neglected its duty in not undertaking research to render opium harmless while preserving its creative attributes.

* *Journal of the American Medical Association*, September, 1971.

Whether belief in ourselves, in a god or in spirits, is induced by drugs, meditation or external stimuli, it is generally agreed that faith in something is an integral part of our lives. Without it few people can live any constructive sort of existence. For many, hope of salvation implies a seeking after perfection in both mind and body, leading to the belief that those who guide us to everlasting life from the next world can demonstrate their existence by healing the afflicted and providing us with good health during our stay in this world.

9

Sickness and Superstition

IN 1832, a great cholera epidemic swept across Europe and eventually reached America. A London dentist wrote a letter to *The Times* urging the government to ring the capital with cannon and fire them off every hour in order to "disinfect the atmosphere."

The notion that noise could neutralize disease was not a new one. Its roots lay in the age-old belief that plagues and epidemics were caused by malevolent spirits, and that they disliked noise and could thus be driven away and their influence ended. In the sixteenth and seventeenth centuries, and even earlier, church bells were often rung when illness ravaged a community, and if they were "fired" or made to clang together instead of ringing in sequence, the beneficial effect would be even greater.

But the cure recommended by the London dentist was not entirely based on superstition. Of the many theories that sought to explain the spread of cholera one of the most popular was that the disease was carried by polluted air. Thus the firing of cannon, or any loud or sudden noise, would disturb the atmosphere and cause the fatal airs to disperse.

In dealing with medical superstitions we face the same problems when trying to assess the healing properties of plants and herbs. The belief or superstition, however bizarre, *may* be based on an element of scientific truth, just as the value of a plant in alleviating symptoms may be due to chemical ingredients quite unknown to the user or prescriber. A further complication may arise when a plant, known to have curative properties, is used not as a medicine, but as an outward symbol or as a means of transferring the disease to another object. We have spoken of the custom of putting a fish into the mouth of a child suffering from whooping-cough and then throwing the fish into

the river. A similar procedure was often used to treat fits and con-
vulsions, when rushes were drawn through the mouth of the patient
and then taken some distance from the house and discarded.

The transference of disease from humans to inanimate objects,
trees and animals, forms a major part of medical folklore. Australian
aborigines sometimes cure toothache with heated stones of a particular
colour and recognizable shape which are then thrown away. In war-
time these stones are collected by tribesmen, who hurl them at their
foes in the hope that they will inherit the toothache and lose the desire
to fight. In Uganda it is common practice for a man suffering from
leg ulcers to rub the afflicted part with the leaves of a certain herb and
then bury the leaves in a footpath. The first traveller to step on the
spot is supposed to acquire the ulcers and the original sufferer will
thus be cured. In Europe the same reasoning is met in the superstition
that to cure a child of croup a young frog must be placed in the
child's mouth and then released in the garden. The child, it is said,
will be cured instantly while the frog will convulsively cough its way
around the garden for many nights to come.

By far the most common objects of disease transference are trees.
There are endless methods of achieving this, from merely running
around the tree (as in Germany) and chanting "God greet thee, noble
tree, I bring thee my gout," to the more painful practice, found in
Hertfordshire, England, of putting one's head against a tree, nailing
a lock of hair to the bark, and then jerking the head away so that
the hair remains on the tree! In Wales it was once the custom to
wash a patient with pieces of rag and then tie them to the branches
of a nearby tree.

Returning to animals, the ancient Irish remedy for whooping-cough
was to pass the child under and over a donkey nine times; this was
probably another belief in disease transference. The domestic cat, too,
has been forced to suffer many indignities in the cause of healing.
One device was to throw the patient's washing-water (or in some
cases the contents of the chamber-pot) over the unsuspecting animal,
upon which it would immediately take to the hills, carrying the disease
with it. For eye afflictions and styes one had to hold a black cat
upside-down and stroke the eye with its tail. For a woman a tom was
required, a queen for a man. Cats were popularly associated with

witches, and feature largely in folklore, representing the powers of both evil and good. The cat's colour is often important, though the powers attributed to it can vary widely from country to country. This is unusual, for one characteristic of all folklore is the consistency with which the same beliefs and superstitions are found all over the world and in very dissimilar cultures. In Britain black cats are considered lucky, but the appearance of a white cat is often held to presage illness and misfortune. In other countries of Europe, and in parts of America, the reverse is true. Fairly common in most countries is the belief that if a cat leaves the house of a sick person and does not return the patient will die. Also widespread is the belief that a sick cat will attract illness to the home; in some areas the sick animal is forcibly ejected and left to its own devices until well again. The abandonment of cats and kittens when moving house is sometimes explained by the superstition that to take a cat to a new house will invite illness or bring disaster.

Superstitions associated with animals in the cure of disease are legion. In some parts of England the froth of the snail was used as a cure for earache, while in Ireland a standard cure for mumps was to lead the patient by a halter three times round a pigsty. Many early medical prescriptions include the dried lungs of a fox as treatment for chest troubles. A Druidic treatment for toothache was the frequent application of dried and calcined bodies of newts. Earlier still Plutarch was singing the praises of the stone-curlew for its ability to cure jaundice merely by staring fixedly at the sufferer. So well known was the bird's power in this respect that bird-merchants of the time used to keep their aviaries covered over in case one bird should inadvertently cure a patient free of charge! The Doctrine of Signatures, the belief that like cured like, applied to animals as much as to plants and herbs. In ancient Greece the gall of eagles was recommended for weak sight as a result of the bird's ability to see over a long distance, and in some countries swallows were eaten regularly for the same purpose. Snail shells were eaten in Tudor times for "fits of the stone." Similarly the bite of a mad dog could be cured by quick application of one of the hairs from the same dog—a custom that has been perpetuated in the expression "a hair of the dog" and has been used by generations of revellers as an excuse for a quick morning drink to cure the hang-over of the night before.

Horse-hairs at one time featured largely in folk-medicine as a cure for worms in children. Once again, imitative therapy is seen to be at work, for the hairs were chopped into short sections resembling thread-worms before being swallowed. Less easy to explain is the ancient schoolboy tradition that a horse-hair held in the hand reduces the pain of a beating. But oddest of all is the widespread belief that the advice of a man riding a piebald horse must be sought as a cure for whooping-cough. The disease itself varies from county to county—the important thing is that the advice of the rider must be followed meticulously, no matter how unlikely it proves to be. A variation of this custom is found in Oxfordshire, where it is used specifically for the cure of goitre. Here the rider must be asked for a hair of the horse's tail, but on no account must be told the reason for the request. Ideally, the horse should be a stallion. One of John Wesley's cures in his *Primitive Physick*, this time for cancer, was to obtain a supply of the hard callous-like "spurs" that grow on the inside of a horse's leg. These should be dried and powdered and administered to the patient in ale and hot milk every six hours.

It is understandable that the birds and animals familiar to country-dwellers should be the object of superstition, and much of it concerned with matters of health. While the "hair of a dog" has traditionally become associated with the effects of excess drinking, a much more venerable remedy to discourage a taste for alcohol was a diet of owls' eggs. This was known to the ancient Greeks, and small boys were given this preparation to ensure that they would not grow up as drunkards. A more practical method of curing alcoholism in medieval times was to slip a live eel into the victim's ale. In effect this was an early form of "aversion therapy."

For centuries in Europe the garden mole has been credited with curing all kinds of complaints. It is particularly associated with the relief of cramp and rheumatism, the forelegs of the animal being carried in the pocket to cure cramp in the arms, the hind legs to cure pain in the lower limbs. A form of transference therapy was to make the mole's nose bleed and let the blood drop on to warts. The animal would then be released and gradually the warts would vanish.

One of the oldest and commonest animal superstitions was that the toad carried in his head a jewel which could be used as an antidote to poison. It could also indicate the presence of toxic substances and in medieval Europe, where the danger of poisoning was ever-present, toad-stones were mounted on rings by those who feared such a death. The stone was said to sweat or grow cloudy in the presence of poisoned food or drink, and one wonders how such an absurd superstition could ever have been taken seriously in view of what must have been a long record of failures. Presumably most of those it failed to protect were in no position to register a complaint. Frogs were also objects of much mystery, though their services were not sought as assiduously as those of toads. But they still had their uses. The dried body of a frog worn in a silk bag round the neck was a sure precaution against epilepsy, and dried frogspawn could be stuffed up the nostrils to combat a nose-bleed.

Dorothy Jacob, in her *Cures and Curses*, describes a particularly unpleasant method of curing the plague which involved a cockerel. The tail feathers of the bird were pulled out and its bare rump thrust into the glowing fire. After frantic struggles the bird would eventually expire, and the process was repeated with a succession of cocks until one finally survived the treatment. At this stage the infection was considered to have left the patient.

In the Blue Ridge Mountains of Virginia, live snails were swallowed as a cure for consumption, and several North American Indian tribes habitually eat snakes to endow themselves with the attributes of speed and deviousness found in the animal.

The power to effect cures was not limited to animals and plants. Metal was well known to have the property of dispelling the forces of evil, and so to cure the disease that had been inflicted. An Irish cure for boils and abcesses was to point the edge of a cutting-tool, or the sharp end of scissors, three times towards the affected part. An opened pair of scissors, forming a cross, was used as a protection against malignant spirits, and could be hidden in a drawer or under a cushion to render harmless the influence of a visitor suspected of being a witch. Knives were also used for this purpose, and were sometimes inserted in a cradle as an alternative to nails to protect the child from illness.

The most common form of metal in circulation was money, and

this was widely used both for protection against disease and as a cure. Most powerful was "sacrament money"—coins given in a church collection and later bought from the priest. The small coins obtained were made into a chain or necklace and were highly valued in many parts of Europe. Sacrament money was particularly useful for treating rheumatism and epilepsy. Its power was greatly enhanced if it had been carried three times round the Communion Table before it left the church. Money also came to be associated with the "royal touch," the healing power attributed to monarchs. In England it seems to have dated from the reign of Edward the Confessor and in France even earlier from the time of Clovis.

The King's Evil, which could be cured by the royal touch, was scrofula, a disease of the bones and joints which often afflicted royalty, and left the victim crippled and deformed. A famous sufferer Dr. Samuel Johnson who, as a child, was brought to London and "touched" by Queen Anne in the last years of her reign. It did little good. Faith in the treatment was declining, for already in the previous reign, William III, with his Dutch dislike of the fanciful, had denounced the custom and tried to end it. On more than one occasion, while reluctantly officiating at the ceremony, he had been heard to express the wish that God would not only heal the sufferers but also put more sense into them!

The hey-day of the royal touch had been a little earlier, in the reign of Charles II (1660–85). Charles was said to have treated more than 100,000 of his subjects at various times. The crowds at the ceremonies were vast and once several people were trampled to death. Apparently this in no way lessened their faith in the treatment, and so the authorities let it be known that the King himself did not need to touch the patient; it was enough if subjects could touch something already handled by the King. Coins were the obvious answer, and in this form the royal touch continued for the rest of the reign.

After Charles died, West Country opposition to the accession of his brother James was centred upon the Duke of Monmouth, Charles' illegitimate son by Lucy Walters. The popularity of the Duke, who had landed at Lyme Regis after several years' exile in France, rose when it was heard that he had cured two cases of the King's Evil since his arrival, at Taunton and at Hinton St. George in Somerset.

The new King, on the other hand, had never cured anyone, though it was known he had tried to. As a result many honest folk in the West of England took this as proof of Monmouth's right to the throne. In the event they paid dearly for their belief, for in 1686, after the Battle of Sedgemoor, nearly three hundred were sentenced to death by Judge Jefferies at the Bloody Assizes and their leader was executed on the order of his uncle, the King. A further sidelight on illness in history is the more recent theory that the savage sentences meted out by Judge Jefferies were due to his lifelong migraine.

The royal touch manifested itself in different ways in different countries. In medieval Denmark the king could cure any childhood disease by touching the infant, while until comparatively recently, in the Tonga Islands, the only disease capable of being cured by this means was scrofula, and that only by the touch of the royal foot.

An ancient myth crediting the king with supernatural powers was that a single look from his eyes could either bless or blight the recipient according to the royal mood. Neither did the king always have to see the person. In the early days of the mikados of Japan the monarch had to sit on his throne staring straight ahead and looking neither to the left or the right. Should he do so, or incline his head in any particular direction, the part of his realm in direct line with his glance would suffer plague, famine or some other calamity. Understandably, successive generations of Japanese royalty expressed their objection to this system, and eventually the crown or some kingly object was placed over the throne as a substitute, leaving the owner free to move about.

The eyes were traditionally held to be the "windows of the soul" and capable of expressing the feelings of a person. Certain people, kings and commoners alike, were thought to have the Evil Eye and could bring disaster upon those they looked at. The Evil Eye was a popular superstition in Europe for centuries and still lingers on in Italy and Sicily. In England it was thought that only the first glance of the day was malevolent, and there is an account of a man in Yorkshire said to be cursed with this characteristic who made sure that his first glance each morning should be directed on a pear tree outside his window, so dissipating its evil influence. The tree, it is said, eventually withered and died. Those possessed of the Evil

Eye had no control over its action, and in some cases were even unaware they had it. The Emperor Napoleon III of France knew himself to have the Evil Eye and wore a talisman on his watch-chain to counteract its effect. In the present century King Alfonso of Spain was thought to have this magical power after a state visit to Italy in 1921 during which several sailors were drowned in mysterious cir-cumstances during a naval review. Pope Leo XIII himself was said to have had the Evil Eye; impressionable Italians pointed to the high mortality rate of cardinals during his pontificate. People with the Evil Eye were feared, and anyone with a squint or wall-eye was considered a great danger. Today, a person finding himself feared and avoided would probably hasten to change his toothpaste or take a course of chlorophyll tablets. But in the days when these modern forms of magic were not available it could turn a normal individual into a recluse, or engender eccentricities that only seemed to confirm the original fears. Quasimodo, the Hunchback of Notre-Dame, with his squint and deformities, is a classic example of how any odd personal feature was associated with magic and witchcraft.

There were, of course, various means of protection from the Evil Eye. The repetition of a prayer, spitting on the ground or crossing the fingers were some. But most powerful of all was extending the first two fingers of the right hand in what later became the Churchillian V-sign. In Europe this gesture had been a form of protection against evil for centuries, and in England had been used for genera-tions by uncultured citizens wishing to express their contempt for law and order—or merely for other citizens. In adapting this famous gesture as a V-for-Victory symbol, Churchill was no doubt fully aware of its ruder implications, for most Englishmen were in no doubt as to the intended destination of the outstretched fingers.

Certain fingers of the hand were also thought to have magical properties. The forefinger of the right hand is sometimes called the Poison Finger and should never be used to spread ointment on wounds or cuts, this function being performed by the longest finger. The third finger of the left hand was supposed to lead directly to the heart, and for this reason became the finger normally used for wedding rings.

Many inanimate objects are supposed to have healing power for reasons which often seem remote. Stones were often used for healing, and if a large stone or rock could be found with a hole in it big enough to accommodate the passage of a sick person, a cure would almost certainly be effected. An example of this belief may still be found in connection with the Long Stone at Minchinhampton, in Gloucestershire. Rocking stones, sometimes called logan stones, were also used in illness, and children would be placed under them in the hope of curing mumps and rickets. In Cornwall, at Nancledra, one such stone was a source of embarrassment when used this way : it refused to rock if the child were illegitimate.

Small stones with holes were sometimes carried on a string or hung over the bed in order to keep rheumatism at bay. Rheumatism is remarkable in being the only illness which a patient can cure by taking a foreign object to bed (a possible exception being infertility!). Sometimes a potato is used, sometimes a small metallic object, especially magnets. But most usually it is a cork from a bottle. This may be placed between the sheets, tied to the leg or held in the hand. Whichever way it is used, thousands are ready to testify to its efficacy in curing cramp to rheumatism. So strong is this belief, in fact, that in 1973 a letter in the august columns of *The Lancet* announced a series of clinical trials connected with the use of bottle corks in bed, using plastic stoppers as a control! The letter was not intended to be taken seriously, but there is little doubt that the results would vindicate the action of bottle corks and leave the stoppers standing, though it is less likely that any logical or scientific reason would be found to account for this phenomenon. Nor is it likely that tests on the wearing of silver or copper rings for the same purpose would reveal any deep scientific truth even when the ring (as is imperative) is made from a coffin-handle.

Many superstitions centre on hospitals and nursing. A common one is that a patient should never be moved feet-first, always head-first, especially when entering the operating theatre. New sheets laid over the back of a chair are an ill omen for the patient and are supposed to portend three successive deaths in the ward. The nurse who finds her apronstrings twisted can expect a change of job, while a patient who knocks over a chair is almost certain to have foreshadowed his own collapse. The bringing of white flowers into wards is rarely welcome. To arrive with a bunch of lilies is tactless in the extreme, as everyone knows these flowers are connected with death. Nobody would be misguided enough to comment on this (except, perhaps, the patient) but after the visitors have gone the offending flowers often vanish without trace. In some hospitals they have a habit of reappearing in the geriatric unit.

At one time no patient was discharged from hospital on a Saturday, for this was thought to be an omen of ill-luck leading to speedy re-admission. Soldiers are notoriously superstitious, especially about battle wounds. Many of these beliefs are still to be found amongst African tribes, and include the custom of finding the arrow that has wounded a warrior, wrapping it in wet rags and keeping it cool. This is thought to stop the wound becoming inflamed, and is a curious parallel with the European belief that to cure a cut one need only wipe the knife with grease, the wound itself requiring no attention.

Many superstitions of soldiers are necessarily of a fatalistic nature, as is the tradition that if a bullet does not have your "number" on it, it will not kill you. Unfortunately, of course, no soldier can know what number is on the next bullet. This same form of comforting fatalism was found amongst many civilians in World War Two when under-going bombing. Equally optimistic was the medieval belief that those who practised sorcery and witchcraft could supply an "ointment of war" that had the power of deflecting weapons.

In seventeenth-century Europe murder by poisoning was an estab-lished art and frequently used to remove relatives who stood between a man and his inheritance. The most common poison in use, arsenic, was sold openly and known as "succession powder." Death by arsenical poisoning was notoriously difficult to diagnose and, in fact, remained the favourite means of murder well into the nineteenth century. In the French and Italian courts of the Middle Ages those who specialized in poisons were careful not to allow their art to become over-simplified. Poisons were divided into three classes accord-ing to the needs of the poisoner. First came the *venena terminata*, poisons which would kill the victim at a predetermined time, according to the customer's instructions. Second were *venena temporanea* which had a slow but steady effect. They would kill eventually, but no time limit was guaranteed. Last were the *venena delibutoria*. These were poisons which killed, not by internal ingestion, but by outward contact. A popular form of poison of this kind was the "perfumed glove" used by Catherine de Medici and said to have been the cause of death of at least one English monarch. Another form of this poison was used in the attempted assassination of the religious and superstitious French monarch Louis XI. An apothecary was paid to supply a liquid which was to be smeared on the corner of the altar, which Louis normally kissed during his devotions. It failed to work, and, as was the custom of those days, the apothecary paid for his failure with his life. What the liquid was we do not know. While arsenic was the favourite form of solid poison, liquids usually consisted of arsenical salts dissolved in nitric acid for external use, or in alcohol for taking internally, often in conjunction with opium.

In witchcraft, murder could be done by sticking pins into a wax image of the victim. Sometimes a sheep's heart or a live toad might be used instead. Insertion of the pins caused illness, but destruction of the image meant death. Today suspicion that a person may be dabbling in witchcraft is more likely to have fatal results for the practitioner. In 1945 the body of Charles Walton, a seventy-four year old hedgecutter, was found in a field in Warwickshire transfixed to the ground by the prongs of a bale fork. His legs and arms were lacerated, presumably in a fight to defend himself, and a rough cross had been slashed on his throat after death. The murderer was never found, though the matter was investigated by Scotland Yard for many months. But they found that Walton had been dabbling in witchcraft all his life and from the age of fifteen had had a name for being able to forecast local deaths. Many thought him a witch, and responsible for local disasters affecting humans and livestock. In 1950 the famous American anthropologist Margaret Mead carried out further investigations into the case and concluded that it was definitely a ritual witchcraft killing. Strangely an almost identical murder had taken place in the village in 1875. Again the victim was suspected of being a witch, and again the murderer was never found. In both cases a conspiracy of silence in the community defeated all efforts to obtain evidence.

Surprisingly there are few superstitions linked with doctors. One of them can be a source of embarrassment, for it is the belief that it is unlucky to pay the doctor's bill in full. The roots of this custom are probably to be found in the old tradition of not telling the gods of one's good fortune lest they destroy it. The implication of not paying all the bill is that medical attendance has not yet ended, and that sickness still surrounds the household. This, too, may be the origin of that most depressing of all medical superstitions—that to admit to feeling well inevitably portends a serious illness!

10

Fringe Medicine

THE term "fringe medicine," coined by Mr. Brian Inglis in 1960 as the title of book, means the treatment of disease by methods based on theories not held by most doctors. Its range is wide and includes homeopathy, acupuncture, osteopathy and chiropractice, as well as various psychiatric techniques, some of which are dealt with elsewhere in this book.

Back to Nature

The basic belief of those who use only herbal medication is that plants contain all we need to cure disease. Medication seems largely unnecessary if the body has been kept in a healthy state by the ingestion of only natural foods. In this context natural foods mean vegetables grown "organically" without the aid of fertilizers and insecticides; they are unadulterated with colouring matter or preservatives and preferably eaten raw. There are many variations on this theme. Some naturopaths claim that vegetables *may* be cooked, as long as the vital juices are not destroyed and the nutritional value remains unimpaired. Others are less interested in natural foods than in natural environment, claiming that the body should be totally exposed to sunlight and fresh air to obtain perfection. The result is the cult of nudism. Combinations of such ideas are found in communities of what were once termed "simple lifers," with their desire to withdraw from the outside world, pool possessions and return to a primitive but healthy way of life.

The "back to Nature" movement represents the oldest form of medical belief. Many doctors subscribe to the belief that, if left alone, Nature will cure most ills. Probably many more are in silent agreement with the aphorism that "the most reliable diagnostic agent is the passage of time." In other words, let the symptoms develop fully before attempting a diagnosis. Most naturopaths believe that by the time symptoms develop the body is well on the road to recovery, without any medication being needed. Others hold that symptoms are not a sign of true illness, but merely demonstrate that the body is taking its own steps to combat a hostile condition. Nature, like Time, is the Great Healer.

There could be a certain amount of danger in this kind of thinking. Presumably those who use slogans like "Nature knows best" are aware that malaria-carrying mosquitos, cancer cells and smallpox virus are also Nature's children. It is hard to see why Nature should prefer to favour mankind rather than the anopholes mosquito or the snails and other disease carriers. The view that Nature will support the human race rather than other forms of life seems on a par with the belief that God is an Englishman, American, or German. One is reminded of the parson who noticed a man tending a well-kept garden. "How wonderful," said he "to see what beauty God and Man can make together." The gardener paused in his digging. "You may well be right, padre," he said, "but you ought to have seen this place when God had it to Himself!"

Many people believe that if God, as Nature, has the human body to itself, it will never ail. Whilst many are content with adopting a diet and a way of life that conforms as closely to this as possible, many others practise it only at times and as a form of medical retreat for the sins of gluttony and excess. Hence the Nature Cure establishments where people hope that two weeks on a diet of natural food will cancel the effect of self-indulgence during the remaining fifty weeks of the year. On the continent of Europe one of the oldest and most famous is the Bircher-Brenner Clinic near Zurich, founded in 1897. In Britain, the Champneys Nature Clinic in Buckinghamshire established a prototype for this kind of treatment during the early 'thirties. Both are still flourishing. Like many others they have attracted the attention of the wealthy and the famous. The resulting publicity has tended to create the impression that few ordinary people can afford a diet of orange-juice and salads, even with massage and osteopathy thrown in. In fact many who attend such clinics do so to slim, often to improve their public image. Most of us eat too much most of the time, and a period of dieting will do no harm. More questionable is the value of natural or organically grown foodstuffs. According to the findings of an American doctor, reported in the *Journal of the American Medical Association* in May 1972, much of what is offered as organically-grown in America is commercially grown and simply sold at 50 to 100 per cent premium. Studies by the U.S. Department of Agriculture show that there is no correlation between fertilizers and nutrients—organically grown fruits and vegetables are *not* more nutritious. In fact, organically-grown products are often poorly shaped, poorly coloured, small, and showing attacks of insects and disease. There is, he adds, not one verified case of an illness caused by pesticide residues on fruit or vegetables bought retail. And lastly, it is unrealistic to think that plants use organic molecules from manure. They can use them only when they have been broken down into inorganic elements dissolved in water.

Bones of contention

Balanced upright on two legs, the human frame is subject to all kinds of strains and stresses. In youth and early manhood these are scarcely apparent as joints and muscles move in a well-oiled and co-ordinated rhythm. Normally not until middle-age do the sudden twinges of backache and the slight stiffening of muscles make one realize that old age is approaching and the machine may need some maintenance.

For centuries the ability of the bonesetter or manipulator to ease these conditions was looked upon as a happy knack, not an orthodox method of treatment. That certain individuals have this skill has long been recognized, but professional recognition has been far longer in coming. Most doctors classed the bonesetter as a quack, but there were exceptions. When Sir Hans Sloane, President of the Royal Society of Physicians, found his niece was suffering from a deformity of the spine he did not seek advice from his medical colleagues, but sent the girl to Mrs. Mapp, the famous bonesetter. Sarah Mapp was one of the most outrageous and flamboyant characters of eighteenth-century London. Repulsive to look at, with an atrocious squint, bloated face and suffering from a hideous eczema (according to the cartoonist George Cruikshank) she had a short, fat body, but enormous strength in her podgy arms, and was a quick and skilful manipulator of bones. She could set a shoulder unaided and gained fame as a mender of broken limbs. Even so she was looked on with suspicion by most doctors, one of whom once sent her a bogus patient to try and catch her out. Mrs. Mapp, who was not easily fooled, soon decided there was nothing wrong with him and suspected a hoax. Her answer was to dislocate the wretched man's shoulder and send him back to his doctor with a message, that if he could not put the matter right, she herself would do it if he returned in a month!

Sir Hans Sloane was one of few physicians to have confidence in Mrs. Mapp. But gradually her skill and public success brought grudging admiration from doctors, and recognition to an art that was to become accepted and known as manipulative surgery. But it was a long battle. Two hundred years later it was still far from being won, and was still raging in the early years of this century when the young and medically unqualified Herbert Barker was gaining fame as a surgical manipulator

The B.M.A. did not approve of Herbert Barker. As he was not a qualified medical practitioner, no disciplinary action could be taken. But they demonstrated their attitude in no uncertain manner when, in 1911, a disciplinary committee struck off Frederick Axham, a doctor who had acted as anaesthetist for Barker.

By 1914 Barker's fame was such that more than fifty Members of Parliament petitioned that he should be allowed to give free treatment to servicemen, as he had requested, but the War Office proved as intransigent as the B.M.A. When he died in 1950, Sir Herbert Barker (he was knighted in 1922) was still medically unqualified, though he had the satisfaction of knowing that his ideas on manipulative surgery were becoming accepted by the medical schools. But Barker was not the originator of osteopathy.

Across the Atlantic, a few years before Barker was born, a country doctor from Virginia named Andrew Taylor Still had become disillusioned with orthodox methods of treatment when his three children died in an outbreak of spinal meningitis. Still studied the structure of the spine and decided that minor disclocations or abnormalities of bone structure contributed to most illnesses, if not actually inducing them. His theory was that good health stemmed from a good flow of blood through the system, which, under normal conditions, built up its own defence mechanism against attacks from disease. Andrew Still argued that malfunction of the joints stopped the flow of blood at that point, and so reduced its ability to produce the chemicals needed to fight illness. The idea that the body will deal with disease in its own way, once complete blood circulation has been restored, is the cardinal precept of osteopathy today. It is the reason why those who practise it claim to cure such afflictions as gallstones, headaches, worms in children, and many other conditions not normally associated with bone structure.

As a form of manipulative therapy, osteopathy has always been viewed with suspicion by the doctors, though it continues to gain converts and is growing in public esteem year by year. Now, at least, doctors send patients to osteopaths openly instead of in the fear of being struck off the register for aiding and abetting an unqualified practitioner. But even the public still think of it in terms of curing backache or lumbago and little else. Few appreciate the relief that osteopathy can bring to sufferers from indigestion and colds, for example. The image of the osteopath as a latter-day Mrs. Mapp still persists.

Another form of manipulation that has some adherents is chiropractice. Here, again, the theory is that the rectification of spinal irregularities (called subluxations) will cure disease, but this time not by allowing better blood circulation but by speeding nerve impulses. Chiropractice is less popular in Britain than in America, where it was founded in the late nineteenth century by Daniel D. Palmer. It was his son, however, who did most to spread the chiropractic gospel by heavy publicity. He developed the idea that the efficiency of the nerves in the spinal cord was directly related to the temperature of the spine at that point. He invented a machine called the neurocalometer which could measure this temperature, and which he hired out to fellow-practitioners for $1,000 down and a similar amount spread over ten years! He followed this with a bigger and better machine, with the unfortunate name of Electroencephaloneuromentimpograph!

Chiropractice, in its early days, had to combat not only the medical profession but the practice of osteopathy, which had begun first. That it has made its present strides in America is partly due to the enthusiasm of the insurance companies. One executive has stated that medical attendance by an orthodox doctor often lasts for weeks or months, with high costs to the company. Yet chiropractors, he maintains, rarely have to attend for more than a fortnight before benefit is felt by the patient.

Curiously, the hostility of doctors to chiropractice has worked in its favour. When Palmer was sent to prison early in his career for treating patients without a medical qualification, to be followed by many other chiropractors up and down the country, it began to look like a vendetta. Public sympathy was aroused, and in the Senate a bill to legalize chiropractice was passed with a huge majority. By 1963 it had been accepted by every state in the Union and in most of them the chiropractor also has the right to sign a death-certificate. The doctors had found—too late—that the best way to put the public on the side of an opponent is to make him a martyr.

Homeopathy

The eighteenth century was noted for human excess. It was also a period of change, when ideas that had been accepted for centuries were soon to be discarded and men like Voltaire, Jean-Jacques Rousseau, John Locke and David Hume began to influence public thinking in a new age of enlightenment.

In medicine, too, changes were imminent. For years doctors had worked on the basis that if a drug worked, then larger amounts of the drug would work even better. As many standard medicines of the pharmacopoeia included such dangerous substances as arsenic and antimony, the number of deaths by poisoning was probably greater than those attributable to the disease.

Here and there doctors expressed their concern about the wisdom of excessive dosage, but few took any action in the matter. One who did was Samuel Hahnemann, a young German doctor from Saxony. His concern was such that, having built up a big practice, he suddenly abandoned it "for fear of doing further injury to the patients." Hahnemann devoted the next few years to a serious study of pharmacology and to the action and effect of drugs and chemicals on the human body. In 1796 he propounded his theory of homeopathy, basing it on the ancient Hippocratic premise that "like cures like."

The idea was an old one, but Hahnemann noted that it had evolved along rather illogical lines. In effect the concept that "like cures like" had been translated into the idea that similarity in appearance or characteristics could cause a plant or a substance to cure disease or bring relief. The eye-bright could cure eye afflictions because its flower resembled the eye; eagle's gall was similarly used to confer the benefit of long sight. Over the years a vast amount of folklore and superstition had grown up, based on an incorrect appreciation of the principle involved.

Hahnemann maintained that the capacity of a plant or drug to cure a condition was nothing at all to do with its outward appearance, but only with its ability to produce the same symptoms as the disease itself, but in modified form. Peruvian bark, for example, used as an antidote for malaria because of its quinine content, was found to induce fever when given to healthy persons. Poisoning from belladonna produced symptoms similar to scarlet fever.

Hahnemann also found that diluting a substance did not reduce its effect, but often increased it. Even when diluted to a point where the drug was scarcely perceptible by analysis it still seemed to exert its therapeutic effect on the body. So began a new and revolutionary concept of medical treatment. As a prophet in his own country, Hahnemann met opposition from the German medical profession. An even greater outcry came from the druggists who saw, in this new form of treatment, their profits from the sale of drugs dwindling away. But in other countries opposition was quickly overcome. In France the fears of doctors were silenced by the President of the Assembly who argued that if homeopathy were nonsense it would soon die a natural death; but that if it were of value, it should be allowed to continue. In Britain an orthodox physician, Harvey Quin, travelled to Germany to receive instruction from Hahnemann himself and returned in 1827 to become the country's first homeopathic practitioner.

Again there was opposition, but Quin was well-connected socially and had treated many members of the aristocracy including Prince Leopold, uncle to the future Queen Victoria. He was a friend of Charles Dickens and William Thackeray and on intimate terms with the colourful Count d'Orsay. Homeopathy quickly became the smart thing of the day and was enthusiastically taken up by the *hautmonde*, most of whom remained blissfully unaware of the theory behind it. Royal interest was not long in coming, and it is from this period that the association between homeopathy and the royal family began. Queen Mary was an enthusiast, as was her son, George VI, who even christened a race-horse Hypericum—the name of a standard homeo-pathic remedy. Royal approval has also shielded homeopathy from the outspoken criticism often faced by other new forms of treatment.

But in early-Victorian times things were different. The fashion of lampooning royalty had reached its height during the Regency and continued well into the era of Victoria and Albert. Quin and his patients were ridiculed by most doctors including influential members of the College of Physicians, one of whom got him blackballed from the Athenaeum Club. Despite this, or perhaps because of it (for the medical profession is slow to learn) more and more doctors began to accept Quin's theories. By 1850 there was enough support to see the establishment of London's first homeopathic hospital at Golden Square, near Piccadilly Circus. By 1870 the *British Homeopathic Pharmacopoeia* was listing all the substances used in homeopathic medicine, the methods of preparing them and the tests required for identification and purity. In America the first such pharmacopoeia was published in Boston in 1897 and there have been several editions since.

Today the principles of homeopathy are accepted by many doctors all over the world. Yet it still plays no part in standard medical train-ing and its adherents are those doctors who have qualified in orthodox medicine and have turned to homeopathy at a later stage. Most doctors still look upon Hahnemann's theories as well-meaning but misguided, though their attitude is slowly changing, especially with the realization of the dangerous side-effects of some orthodox drugs today. Yet it remains a paradox that in Britain, where the beginnings of homeopathy seemed so auspicious, its standing is far lower than in other countries such as Germany and France. This may be due to the care which British homeopathists have always taken to remain respectable and their insistence that homeopathic treatment should be practised only by qualified doctors and not by laymen. Unfortunately

this has resulted in an apparent rigidity of attitude, for the homeopathic practitioner remains first and foremost a doctor of medicine,
with the innate conservatism of his profession. His views remain as
rigid about homeopathic medicine as they do about orthodox medicine, and in this framework progress seems unlikely.

Acupuncture and pulse doctrine

The practice of acupuncture is founded on the ancient Chinese belief
that certain points on the body are directly connected with the internal
organs, and that these organs can therefore be affected by external
stimuli at these points. Pain may be reduced this way, and the organ
energized or sedated according to the type and degree of malfunction.

The points, called acupuncture points, are divided symmetrically
throughout both halves of the body and number approximately 700.
In addition, points on widely separated parts of the body are connected to the same internal organ, and connected between themselves
on the surface by meridians. Meridians also exist connecting points
between other parts of the skin as well as with muscle.

Where osteopathy seeks to stimulate the flow of blood through the
system, and chiropractice claims to transmit nerve impulses, acupuncture speeds energy from the point to the organ concerned. The impulse
is transmitted to the brain and then back to the diseased organ, and
so restores its balance.

To understand the meaning of balance in this context it must be
appreciated that Chinese philosophy was based on the belief in *Yin*
and *Yang*—the division of everything into two opposing elements.
Yin represented all that was negative (dark, cold and feminine) and
Yang all that was positive (light, warm and masculine). In medicine
this theory was applied to the organs of the body. These were classified into active and passive groups, corresponding to Yang and Yin.
The grouping is as follows :

Active "working" Yang organs	*Passive "storage" Yin organs*
large intestine	lungs
stomach	spleen
Small intestine	heart

Active "working" Yang organs	*Passive "storage" Yin organs*
urinary bladder	kidneys
gall bladder	liver

By inserting tiny needles into the points on the meridian, the flow of energy could be stimulated or controlled, and the organ brought back into the correct balance according to its classification.

As acupuncture has persisted in China for almost 5,000 years it might seem presumptuous to call it Fringe Medicine. The reason for this is that in the west it has only recently aroused interest, though as far back as 1893 the British neurologist Sir Henry Head found that diseased organs could produce pain in other parts of the body far removed from the site of the illness. Even more important was the discovery that if these sites of pain were heated or massaged, the condition of the organ sometimes improved. Since 1950 more attention has been paid to these findings and the growing alarm at the side-effects of much orthodox medicine has stimulated the demand for new forms of treatment. As an indication of this, the magazine *Woman's Own* is said to have received more than 10,000 enquiries from readers after printing a short article on acupuncture.

One can scarcely write off a form of treatment that has been used successfully for so long, yet it has been slow in penetrating the west. Perhaps it was because of lack of communication (the first serious treatise on acupuncture did not appear in Europe until 1863) coupled with resistance to what must seem to western eyes a most peculiar method of treatment. But then so many oriental ideas seem odd to western ears, yet how logical many of them are! What could be more sensible than the Chinese custom of paying the doctor only when the patient is well? Under this system he has every incentive to keep his patients healthy, a custom leading to a greater concern with preventive medicine and less with devising new curative techniques. For this reason personal attention by Chinese doctors continues all the time, during health as well as sickness, and has given rise to methods of early diagnosis that do not unduly interrupt the normal life of the patient.

Of these methods by far the most important is diagnosis by pulse, a technique almost as old as acupuncture. Western procedure is to take the pulse by feeling the radial artery at the wrist. It provides information about the rhythm and frequency of the heartbeat and the condition of the aortic valves. Chinese doctors take the pulse not only at the wrist but at several other points including the neck and legs. Again, where western doctors merely satisfy themselves on the speed and comparative strength of the pulse, Chinese doctors attach the utmost importance to the degree of pressure used to diagnose a condition. A publication of the Chinese Academy of Traditional Medicine (Pekin, 1959) lists twenty-eight different degrees of pressure used in diagnosis, and also differentiates between the various fingers used in this technique. Since World War Two attempts have been made to assess the accuracy of diagnosis by this means. One of the most recent tests was between French doctors and their Chinese colleagues. In 80 per cent of the cases the finding of the doctors coincided, although the Chinese had made their diagnosis by pulse only. Orientals are certainly known to have more sensitive fingertips than westerners, but, like acupuncture, there is clearly something here that needs more study in the west.

Yet another aspect of oriental medicine is moxibustion, in which small cones are placed on the skin and ignited as a treatment for internal disorders. This form of therapy is more widespread than acupuncture, and as a form of counter-irritant has long been known in the western world. The western equivalent of moxibustion took the form of blisters induced by heat or chemicals as a means of stimulating the flow of blood, a practice that died out only at the end of the nineteenth century. But in primitive tribes it still finds favour, and the Ohama Indians of America to this day treat stomach pains by pushing the stem of the shoestring plant into the skin near the site and setting fire to it.

Fringe medicine includes many other methods of diagnosing and healing that seem to work—auto-suggestion, hypnosis, diagnosis of disease by watching the action of a pendulum. It is easy to ridicule them, particularly as they often lend themselves to trickery and commercial exploitation. Those that are palpably false are short-lived. But others have a history going back many centuries with a hard core of success that defies the passage of time. Just as herbs and plants proved efficacious for reasons unknown to the users, perhaps atomic energy research will provide an understanding and proof of many things too easily pushed aside as illogical or unscientific. We do not yet understand how some things work, but this is no reason to deny their existence, any more than it would be reasonable for a savage to deny the existence of radio or photography. There is evidence that some scientists, at least, are now moving to this point of view.

11

Taking the Cure

"ONE would think the English were ducks; they are forever waddling to the waters," remarked Horace Walpole in 1790. If society in England thronged to spas and watering places it was not the only country where this was happening. On the continent such places were even more abundant, for the tradition of the public bath, popularized by the Romans and inherited from the Greeks, had never been forgotten as had happened during the Dark Ages in Britain.

The ancient town of Vichy was already famous for its alkaline springs when it was sacked by the Normans in the ninth century. Charlemagne himself held councils of war in the great marble bath he had built at Aachen, filled with the sulphurous waters well known to the Romans. Further south, on the banks of the Danube, the little town of Pest had been visited for a thousand years by pilgrims eager to bathe in its hot and healing springs.

In Britain the most famous centre had been at Bath. But the departure of the Romans had obliterated the memory of this watering place and it remained hidden and in ruins until rediscovered in the fourteenth century. Even then it was another four hundred years before Bath emerged into its former glory.

The Middle Ages in England saw the gradual emergence of various holy wells and springs whose curative powers were attributed to the saints or to the Virgin Mary. These places became centres of pilgrimage and a useful source of revenue to the Church. Occasionally the diocesan authorities became jealous of the wealth accumulated by a small parish in this way and tried to divert it to their own needs. This happened at North Marston, Buckinghamshire, whose famous holy well was associated with the miracles performed by a former priest, the Blessed John Schorne, whose bones were preserved in the church. In 1456 it was decided to move these relics to Windsor and North Marston ceased to be a place of pilgrimage. Yet faith in its healing powers did not die, and well into the present century sufferers from gout and rheumatism were still taking the waters. The value of the waters was also noted by local doctors and druggists who, during the seventeenth century, would come at night to the well and bottle the waters ready to sell in their dispensaries the next day.

The Reformation in England saw the suppression of many of these supposedly miraculous springs, and a century later the Commonwealth further discouraged their use. Even so it was recognized that their powers, even if not miraculous, were still real and depended to a large extent on the mineral content of the water.

In Europe one of the best-known mineral springs was at Spa, in the Belgian Ardennes, a place that eventually gave its name to this kind of watering place. It was an iron, or chalybeate, spring that provided the waters and attracted patients from all over Europe. Another famous spa was at Baden, Switzerland, and in the years that followed many such places grew into fashionable resorts patronized by royalty and high society and perpetuated in names such as Gastein, Ems, Pyrmont, Baden Baden, Contrexeville, Marienbad, Homburg and Apollinaris.

In the seventeenth century the fame of these continental spas spread to England and caught the attention of those who saw their commercial possibilities. The rise of several obscure villages into fashionable resorts can be traced from this period; there was Tunbridge Wells (1606), Scarborough (1622), Epsom (1625), Sadlers Wells (1683), Islington (1685), and Cheltenham (1716). Later came Droitwitch, Harrogate, Leamington, Malvern and Matlock, with Llandrindod in Wales and Moffat and Strathpeffer in Scotland.

From the 1740s America, too, began to exploit various springs and wells used by the Indians such as Berkeley Spring, Virginia; Saratoga, Bedford Spring in Pennsylvania, Gettysburg, Buffalo and Poland Spring, Maine.

At most spas, whether in Europe or America, the value of the treatment depended on the chemical content of the water. Some, like Spa itself or Tunbridge Wells, were rich in iron, giving the water its characteristic rusty appearance. At others the water was salty, betraying the presence of the soluble chlorides and sulphates of magnesium, sodium and calcium, as at Homburg and Woodhall Spa in Lincolnshire. Some spas were noted for the presence of carbonic acid gases and sulphuretted hydrogen, producing the evil-smelling fluids eagerly swallowed at Harrogate, Baden and at the famous American spa at White Sulphur Springs in West Virginia. At many places, including Bath itself, the healthful properties of the water depended not on their mineral content but on their purity or comparative warmth. At a fairly late stage the cult of cold water for its own sake was fostered at Grafenburg in the Austrian Alps; it was also seen in England at Malvern where patients who had tried all other forms of therapy became desperate enough to submit to a diet consisting almost entirely of glasses of cold water, which they drank wrapped in nothing but wet sheets!

Such measures seem extreme, yet they were no more fanciful than some of the claims made for the curative powers of spring water. As far back as 1567 the celebrated Dr. Turner, a pioneer of "the cure," was recommending the waters of Bath for :

> *The puffing uppe of the legs with winde;*
> *The madness called Melancholie;*

and

> *The vayne appetite of going to the stoole when*
> *a man can do nothing when he commeth there.*

This frustrating experience dogged many who took the waters, and had been the main reason for Epsom's short-lived fame as a spa, though it gave its name to one of the most famous purgatives of all time—Epsom Salts.

John Wesley, an ardent advocate of natural healing, was keen about the healthful properties of pure water. He recommended cold baths for deafness, blindness and the falling sickness. "One apparently dead from being struck by lightning" could be revived by immediate immersion in cold water, while raging madness could be cured by making the patient wear a hat filled with snow for three weeks.

As ever, many charlatans were ready to cash in on the craze for cures by water and in 1750 a certain Matthew Chancellor claimed to have had a dream in which a spring near his home at Glastonbury had suddenly cured his asthma. Before long asthmatics and others were arriving at Glastonbury at the rate of two thousand a week and Matthew was doing a roaring trade in the spring which he sold locally and sent in bottles to London for sale in the Strand. But it was not to last. A London evening newspaper conducted an analysis, and the water was found to be no different from that in a hundred other springs round the countryside.

Despite the belief that "taking the waters" was a cure-all, the daily routine at a spa involved much more than drinking glasses of water and taking a daily dip. Strict instructions were given by resident physicians, and patients warned to allow a full fifteen minutes before one glass of water and the next, the intervening time to be taken up in "agreeable conversation." Spas were used mainly by the wealthy with time on their hands, and by those trying to repair the damage of a profligate life. The object was to slow the tempo of life, to adjust to a more relaxed and contemplative existence, and to take gentle exercise and gaze on beautiful surroundings between whiles bathing langorously in the beneficial waters. All kinds of additional treatments were on sale. There were steam baths, rain baths, baths of pine and lavender, as well as many aspects of massage, known then as "champooing." The patient could be scalded for half an hour by near-boiling water from a hose or sprayed with ice-cold water from a shower. Some spas supplied mud baths and, incredible as it may seem, one hydro sat its patients in a bath of freshly-prepared and steaming tripe!

Towards the end of the eighteenth century there developed an interest in the inhalation of certain gases and in 1798 Dr. Thomas Beddoes opened his Pneumatic Institute for Relieving Disease by Medical Arts at Clifton, near Bristol. The basis of pneumatic medicine (as it was called) was the idea that ordinary air, consisting of nitrogen and oxygen, was chemically changed in the lungs and became almost pure oxygen. In 1767 Joseph Priestley had discovered carbon dioxide and went on to discover more gases produced by the action of heat or acid on metals and vegetable substances. Carbon dioxide was claimed to cure several diseases, and a Dr. Hey of Leeds used it in cases of tuberculosis and thought his patients much improved. Dr. John Ewart of Bath treated two cases of breast cancer with the gas by applying it directly to the affected parts and said one patient had been completely cured.

After Dr. Beddoes had formed his Institute, with equipment specially designed by the famous engineer, James Watt, other gases were used including pure oxygen and nitrous oxide. Beddoes soon needed a full-time assistant. He chose a young Cornishman, Humphrey Davy, whom he put in charge of the laboratory to conduct research on the properties of gases. Davy found that nitrous oxide not only gave a feeling of euphoria when inhaled but also seemed to lessen sensitivity to pain. Though Pneumatic Medicine had vanished into thin air by the middle of the next century it was the experiments of Humphrey Davy that laid the foundations of modern anaesthesia.

Electricity, too, played its part as an adjunct to the beneficial effects of taking the waters, the two were often combined in a highly dangerous manner. The retiring rooms of many spas were festooned with wires and dotted with dials, all intended to reduce symptoms and provide renewed health. Electrodes were applied to the spine to reduce stiffness, and electric heat was brought into play in the treatment of kidney trouble, high blood-pressure and cardiac conditions. At Smedley's Hydro, at Matlock, Derbyshire, constipation was cured by the simple expedient of inserting a live electrode into the anus, a process graced with the title of "rectal Faradization."

While treatment was not confined to the use of water, life at a spa did not consist entirely of treatment. Even with exercise, vapour-baths, mud baths and massage there were many leisure hours to fill each day. If Bath and other watering places were to compete with their continental rivals they had to provide comparable amenities and entertainment. So far seventeenth-century spas in England had provided entertainment mainly for the local inhabitants. Mixed bathing in the nude by young and old was a normal practice, watched with interest by the assembled company, and Ned Ward, writing about Bath in 1700, hinted strongly at some of the things that went on below the murky surface of the waters. Everything was, if not exactly decorous, at least leisurely. Splashing about in the water was frowned upon, for lady bathers had their toiletries and cosmetics floating on trays near them while they immersed themselves. As soon as they left they put on voluminous red cloaks before retiring to the vapour rooms or other treatment rooms.

Some spas, including Bath and Carlsbad, were said to induce fertility, though the more cynical writers of the period attributed the many pregnancies more to the local gallants than to the action of the waters.

At Bath, the arrival of Richard ("Beau") Nash in 1705 brought some order into the chaos that existed. Nash, a well-known gambler and rake, was appointed assistant to the Master of Ceremonies in that year, but on the death of his superior in a duel a few months later, was promoted to take his place. He at once displayed a hidden talent for administration and an expertise at fund-raising and publicity.

He began by inviting subscriptions from the wealthy, and with the money raised put on music in the Pump Room, improved the accommodation, opened a theatre, coffee shops, and reading and writing rooms. But as well as all this, Nash imposed strict rules to raise the standard of behaviour not only in the baths but wherever visitors congregated.

His flair for publicity was seen in the daily publication of a list naming new arrivals and stating at which hotel they were staying. For the most important visitors the abbey bells were rung from the moment of their appearance on the outskirts of the town until they had reached their lodgings, outside which they were serenaded by the town band. All this had to be charged for, but, though some objected, most were flattered at the attention paid to them and paid up with good grace. Nash grew rich.

Yet, during his reign of over forty years as Master of Ceremonies at Bath, Nash was not entirely concerned with making money for himself. Much of the revenue was spent on improving the roads in and around the city, in organizing regular cleaning of the baths and surrounding rooms, and installing illuminations and lighting. Nash also felt strongly that the poor should not be denied the benefits of the waters and, with the famous Dr. Oliver, founded a free water-hospital for the poor at Bath which today is the Royal National Hospital for Rheumatic Diseases.

A professional gambler himself, Nash ensured that the gaming tables were run with absolute fairness. Anyone caught cheating was run out of town immediately, with full publicity. Yet more than once Nash paid the debts of an honest but unlucky gambler who could not meet his commitments. In time gambling, whoring, seduction and match-making were carried on so much that the medical aspect of a stay in Bath became the least of its attractions. Daniel Defoe, visiting Bath in 1722, felt sure that the number of sick people taking the cure was only a small fraction of those attending, and that most enjoyed the best of health. Indeed, so notorious did Bath become that in 1735 John Wesley opened a revivalist campaign there, determined (as he put it) "to attack Satan in his headquarters." Alarmed at the effect this might have on his clientele, Nash tried to stop Wesley, but soon recognized that he had met his match. He did not try again, and in the years that followed Wesley and other preachers thundered against vice and Godlessness in the Methodist chapel provided by the Countess of Huntingdon.

Nash himself, though a born administrator, was also a most colourful personality and wit. His sobriquet of "Beau" was not earned for nothing, and he was famous for the sumptuousness and impeccability of his attire. The aristocracy might laugh at him behind his back, but they feared his caustic wit. On one occasion an ancient and wealthy countess who was not popular with Nash, and who was bent almost double with arthritis, announced gushingly that she had come straight from London to see him. "In that case," said the Beau, "you've become damnably warped on the way!"

Meanwhile, in the rest of Europe, the longer-established spas at Vichy, Borège, Forges, Carlsbad, Baden and countless other places where enjoying equal prosperity. Madame de Sevigné went to Vichy several times. She recorded her dislike of fashionable women who insisted on dressing up to be ill. Aix-la-Chapelle, long famous for its hot baths and sweat-chambers, was popular with the aristocracy whose behaviour (according to a contemporary) was enough to make anyone a republican. Peter the Great of Russia went to Spa when in need of relaxation, where he drank twenty-one glasses of water a day and attracted much publicity, all of which was of benefit to the little town. Soon Spa became known as the Café of Europe, and an essential port-of-call for those on the Grand Tour. Even Casanova found it profitable to dally there, though (as he recounts in his

Memoirs) even he was shocked at the improper suggestions made to him by an elderly English dowager!

During the nineteenth century European spas grew more and more fashionable. In England, Leamington, Harrogate and Buxton were flourishing, and from time-to-time a new spa was opened in the hope that it would in turn become fashionable. At tiny Dorton, in the heart of rural Buckinghamshire, a spa was opened in 1834 centred on a sulphurous spring found in a copse at the bottom of Brill Hill. A company was formed to promote the venture. A magnificent building and assembly room were planned, with three orchestras in constant attendance. For a few years the quality flocked to Dorton, though the building was not yet complete, and at last it was announced that Queen Victoria herself would come to take the cure. Alas, it was not to be! Unaccountably the Queen changed her mind and went to Leamington instead. Society dropped Dorton like a hot brick, and today its brief glory can be traced only in the depths of a dense wood where crumbling masonry, almost hidden in the undergrowth, indicates the outline of the former buildings. But a brick-built well still produces the evil-smelling brew that so many came to drink, and, sniffing it today, one can perhaps understand the Queen's decision to take the cure elsewhere.

There were certainly plenty of other places available during Victorian times and an 1895 guide book lists nearly thirty of them. Unfortunately few were favoured by royalty, who seemed to prefer the delights of France and Germany. The Prince of Wales led the fashionable world with constant visits to Homburg and Baden Baden and later, as Edward VII, to Carlsbad and Marienbad. But with the passing of King Edward and the advent of World War One the English spa suffered a death blow from which it never recovered.

Despite a certain loss of prestige amongst continental spas, many of them flourish to this day. To some extent this is due to the differing attitude of the continentals. In England one took the cure (at least in theory) when one was actually ill. But abroad a family would make an annual expedition to a favourite spa irrespective of their state of health. This still applies in most of Europe, and today, while Bath is virtually the sole example of its kind in England, France and Germany between them can still boast nearly four hundred active spas. The Soviet Union has another three hundred or so, mainly on the Black Sea.

Another reason for the decline of the spa in Britain can be found in the rise of the seaside resort as a health cure and tonic for jaded nerves and physique. Whilst the cure in Europe became intimately associated with inland spas, the long and convoluted coastline of Britain lent itself to the establishment of innumerable watering-places where water was available in far greater quantity than from a spring or two. Yet the rise of the seaside resort in England came about almost by accident. It dates from a day in 1626 when a certain Mrs. Farrow, picking her way along the beach at Scarborough, suddenly spied a spring of a curious colour spilling its water down the cliff face. She noticed a patina of rusty red on the rocks on which it fell. Mrs. Farrow, who was evidently of an enquiring nature, sampled the water and found it did her good. She told others of her find and in the months that followed many local residents, and others from far afield, beat a path to the spring and took home bottles of the reddish water. What Mrs. Farrow had found was not all that rare. It was a chalybeate, or iron, spring, just like the springs that made the fortunes of Harrogate and Tunbridge Wells. But the great difference was that Scarborough's spring was by the sea, a fact used by a local physician, Dr. John Wittie, to publicize the place. Dr. Wittie's theory was that if the spring waters of Scarborough were valuable medicinally, the same might well be true of the seas that washed its beach. And so announcements began to appear proclaiming the value of the sea at Scarborough as a valuable tonic, and as a cure for most ailments when taken internally.

By 1753 the town was well known, but as yet only as a centre of the sick and ailing. The idea that the seaside could be a source of pleasure had not yet arrived, and the first boarding houses to be built on the cliffs all faced inland !

Dr. Wittie's attempt to convince the public that the sea around Scarborough was uniquely healthful could not last long. Other seaside villages began to make similar claims, though not so blatantly as Scarborough, and by the end of the century a few within easy reach of the metropolis had achieved some notoriety. Chief among these was Brighton, on the Sussex coast, and a convenient fifty miles from London.

To Brighton, in 1783, came the young Prince George for the first time, brought by his uncle the Duke of Cumberland who thought he needed a rest from life in the capital. The Prince found Brighton to his liking, small though it was, with enough interest and amenities to make it a pleasant change from London. He came again, and again, and in 1785 Brighton received the royal accolade when "Prinny", as he was known, bought a plot of land in the town and decided to build himself a private residence. His first house was undistinguished, but twenty years later there arose on the site the monstrous and bizarre domes and minarets of the Royal Pavilion, designed by Nash. They are there still, a permanent reminder of an extraordinary era and in no small degree responsible for Brighton's slightly raffish and unreal air that has remained as a legacy of Regency days.

But while Brighton remains for ever linked with the Prince Regent it was not the only seaside town to enjoy royal favour. The year after the Prince first visited Brighton his father, George III, had spent some time at Weymouth, and later other members of the royal family were to honour Worthing and Southend in the same way. Gradually it became the custom for those with time and money to spare to spend a week or two each year by the sea, dutifully bathing from the wheeled machines provided and in the care of the professional dippers. Bournemouth began its aristocratic ascent in 1810 and thirty years later was described as "the favoured retreat of the invalid." In its pine-clad setting sheltered from the winds, Bournemouth was indeed beneficial to invalids. Almost too beneficial, in fact, for once in residence they practically refused to die. They settled there in old age, the wealthy and the titled, and gave to Bournemouth the genteel and cataleptic atmosphere that was to mark it out from other resorts. Typically, when the railways came, Bournemouth refused to be associated with such a vulgar invention, and the line skirted the town and provided the nearest station at Poole, five decent miles away.

In other seaside towns the railway had had more effect. Margate, Ramsgate, Hastings were all growing popular, and in Lancashire Blackpool was becoming the holiday centre of the industrial North.

By the end of the century holidays for working people were more common, and the medicinal and therapeutic effect of the "marine fluid" was largely forgotten. No longer did folk drink sea water, and when they bathed it was for pleasure and not as a cure. And so it has remained. Yet even today the tonic properties of the seaside are not quite forgotten, for a change of scenery and a lungful or two of what is popularly described as ozone are still considered to be as beneficial as the sulphur springs of Baden or the waters of Buxton or Harrogate.

While the aristocracy and society flocked to take the waters in the eighteenth century there was little incentive for the rest of the country to drink water in any form. Most urban supplies were polluted and the drink of the ordinary citizen was beer. The middle classes drank French and Spanish wine. Then, as today, the balance of payments exercised the mind of the government, and in 1690, in an attempt to curb imports of foreign wines, a heavy tax was imposed on them. But in addition it was decided to remove the duty on spirits and to allow anyone to distil them without licence.

The effect was immediate and disastrous. In the years that followed England became a nation of drunkards, and the lurid illustrations of William Hogarth and others indicate the terrible depravity that was reached when the poor found spirits within their grasp. This was the era of the gin shop, with its promise to make customers "drunk for a penny, dead-drunk for tuppence." Despite the re-imposition of duty on gin in 1729 and a ban on distillation in 1736, the damage was done. As happened later in America during the days of Prohibition the industry merely went underground, and it was not until the end of the century that the situation began to improve. The effect of gin and spirits generally had not only damaged the nation's health but also resulted in a slackening of morals and general standards of be- haviour. Towards the end of the century various associations were formed for the Improvement of Manners, and though they were aimed chiefly at the flood of pornographic literature they also hoped to reduce drunkenness.

The first years of the nineteenth century saw the formation of associations devoted entirely to the suppression of strong drink, first in Ireland and Scotland, and finally in England. The original aims of such societies were to wean the working man away from spirits, but still allow the drinking of wine and beer. Hogarth himself had tried to do this in his drawings of the depravity and vice in *Gin Lane* compared with the civilized behaviour of those drinking in *Beer Alley*. The first Temperance Society in England was formed at Bradford early in 1830 and the movement quickly spread during the year to Manchester, Birmingham, Leeds and Bristol. It came to London in November.

The early years of the Temperance movement were marked by frequent arguments and opposition both from those who thought the aim should be total abstention from alcohol, and from others, like the breweries and publicans, who argued that there should be no propaganda against the sale of liquor of any kind. Oddly enough, despite the medical evidence of the dangers of prolonged drinking, the medical profession itself raised almost as much objection to Total Abstinence as did the brewers. As it happened the movement against alcohol began just when doctors were beginning to sing praises of alcohol as a medicine, and when hundreds of patent medicines exerted their effect mainly by their high alcoholic content. For this reason those who "signed the pledge" in those early days found a loophole in the clause "except medicinally" when promising to abstain from alcohol. The famous Irish propagandist, Father Matthew, remarked that he had no idea that a man who signed the pledge might have a doctor's certificate in his pocket allowing him to drink alcohol, and soon deleted this clause from the form of promise signed. Many examples were given of people who had become alcoholics from drinking medicine, and alcohol was blamed for the rapid spread of cholera in England from 1832. One classic story told of a man who had been prescribed brandy to cure a serious illness and who had died from delirium tremens six months later.

The first physician to embrace the cause of Total Abstinence was the twenty-three year old Dr. Ralph Grindrod of Manchester who signed the pledge in 1837. But few members of his profession held such views for long, and most of the medical evidence against alcohol was still propagated by well-meaning laymen.

The fantastic stories claiming to show the evils of drink were easily disproved by the doctors. Typical was the tale that a heavy drinker might burst into flames if he stood near a gas jet or lit a match. Even Charles Dickens, in *Bleak House*, describes the death by spontaneous combustion of an alcoholic junk merchant. When challenged on the point, Dickens quoted several cases he had heard of in America, including the dramatic incident when a drunken traveller, warming himself by the fire in a railway waiting room, suddenly fell to the floor with jets of blue flame issuing from his ears, mouth and nostrils.

Much of the opposition of doctors to Total Abstinence sprang from their notorious tenderness about being told what they should and should not prescribe. Until recently, their tenderness has constantly stood in the way of medical progress. But even if the more lurid stories about the effects of alcohol could be discounted, real harm was done to a family when wages went on drink. In time, doctors began to sympathize with those who advocated teetotalism. This curious name came from the famous speech of Dicky Turner, a reformed drunkard, at Preston in 1833. Turner had been voicing his contempt for those who advocated "moderation" in alcohol, and, working himself up into a fury, roared: "I'll have nowt to do with this moderation; I'll be reet down and out tee-tee-total for ever!" And teetotal the movement became in the public mind, though many still used the word Temperance to cover all forms of teetotalism, to the annoyance of those who were in favour of total abstinence. Many doctors who were converted to the cause made statements as wild and unscientific as the laymen before them. One London surgeon announced that "alcohol is a poison," and gave the movement a slogan that has lasted to this day.

Many were the alternatives to alcohol sought as a relief from pain including peppermint, camomile tea, camphor water and the curious "temperance brandy"—a pinch of cayenne pepper in boiling water. The most famous medical advocate of teetotalism in the late-Victorian era was the surgeon Sir Victor Horsley. With Dr. Mary Sturge, he published various works describing the fatal effect of alcohol on plants and animals. One such experiment, in which vegetables were proved to wither and die after being watered with a weak solution of alcohol, was seized on by an anti-abstinence doctor, C. A. Mercier, and ridiculed in his own writings. Mercier promised that no longer would he water his cabbages with Mouton Rothschild or '47 port, as this was obviously a waste. But as sewage was held to benefit plants he assumed that Horsley, if he were consistent, would urge the eating of sewage by his patients to maintain good health. Other eminent doctors, less caustic, reminded their colleagues that Louis Pasteur's work on antiseptic surgery was a direct result of his study of alcohol in a brewery, and in 1882 a Dr. William Sharpe commented that "The stimulus of alcohol, when judiciously controlled, always leads to higher mental effort . . ."

Oddly enough the teetotal movement also met opposition from churches and chapels, many of whom took alcohol as part of their services, or as part of the tradition of induction to the clergy. In the Presbyterian Church the minister "sealed the gown" with a bottle of wine when ordained, and was "fined" a bottle of wine by his colleagues if he had a sermon published or moved into a new manse. St. Paul's comment (1 *Timothy* v, 23) that "a little wine" should be taken to cure infirmities was often quoted to prove that teetotalism was heretical if not positively blasphemous, and in the early days of the movement its adherents were classified as atheists and chapel doors closed to them. So strong was this feeling that in South Shields in the 1840s the noncomformist chapels banded together with the publicans and doctors and hired gangs of toughs to break up teetotal meetings. Even Cardinal Manning, who signed the pledge in 1872, insisted that total abstinence was a sin. He maintained that any man who said that the use of wine in itself was sinful was "a heretic, condemned by the Catholic Church."

Today, though the nonconformists have largely adopted total abstinence, the Catholic Church still take the view that there is nothing sinful about drinking if done in moderation. The sight of devout Catholics coming out of church on Sunday mornings and repairing immediately to the Catholic Club next door for a lunchtime drink is viewed with horror by most nonconformists. However. many impartial observers consider this an improvement on the system once operating in Wales and other nonconformist centres when worshippers ostentatiously dispersed after service only to meet again later at the back door of the local inn. Since Sunday opening in South Wales this custom has virtually ceased, though once it did much damage to the Nonconformist cause.

Today, the medical profession is neither strictly pro- nor anti-alcohol, but the use of spirits as medicine has more or less ended. Oddly enough a relic still lingers in retail pharmacy, where the sale of wines can be allowed by virtue of a "Medicated Wine Licence." Unfortunately just what constitutes a medicated wine has never been established, and in law there is no provision for such a licence.

Today a pharmacist applying for a medicated wine licence is granted a full off-licence, but is trusted to sell only medicated wines, mainly Phosferine or Sanatogen Tonic Wine or similar brands containing small quantities of hypophosphites or quinine. For years one of the best-selling wines in most pharmacies with a medicated wine licence was Gilbey's Invalid Port, which contained no medication at all, and sold entirely on the strength of its name.

In the light of increased knowledge on the depressant effect of alcohol, doctors no longer prescribe stout and porter (so called because it was once the staple diet of Dublin market porters), nor do they urge their patients to drink several glasses of wine a day. In certain cases, however, spirits are still prescribable under the National Health Service. This occasionally happens in the terminal stages of diseases such as cancer or tuberculosis, where gin or whisky is prescribed in conjunction with cocaine or morphine according to the famous recipe of the Brompton Hospital.

12

Death and Superstition

IN the later nineteenth century, discussion of sex was virtually taboo. Today, a century later, it is death which must never be mentioned.

Yet throughout the ages mankind has been obsessed with the inevitability of death, and his inability to lift even a corner of the curtain that separates this world from the next. The lack of knowledge that surrounds the hereafter—if there is one—has created a vast and fearful accumulation of superstition and conjecture, much of it concerned with the spirits of the departed and their possible influence on the living.

Despite a persistent lack of evidence to support it, belief in an after-life has continued since the beginning of time. Many ancient cultures, such as the Egyptians, believed that life in the world to come was much like life on earth; and so the departed was furnished with food and drink to sustain him on his journey and for use in the next world. Oriental religions, on the other hand, tended to the belief that future existence was rebirth in this world, with more or less happiness according to the individual's behaviour. The Christian Church spread the gospel of a purely spiritual world, with purgatory or hell as a temporary or permanent punishment for the sinful. Yet it is rare to find any culture that welcomed contact with the souls of the dead, and many feared it. The Christian Church, for the most part, actively discouraged it, believing that no good could come of interference in matters that have never clearly been understood.

Many superstitions about death have lived into modern times, even though their roots are buried in the past. While everything was done to keep an ailing person alive, for example, it sometimes became obvious that no more could be done. On such occasions, the family would hasten the departure of the person's soul, and in rural localities as late as the nineteenth century physicians were often faced with a death which, though obviously imminent, caused some surprise at its suddenness. A favourite means of procuring "a happy release" was suddenly to snatch the pillow from behind the head of a dying person and let the head jerk back. Another method was to tie a wide tape around the dying man's neck and slowly tighten it until life departed. The kindly countrywoman who thus speeded the departure of her spouse would have been troubled and bewildered at the suggestion that murder had been committed, and few country doctors were tactless enough to suggest it.

Once the person had died, it was essential that nothing should hinder the flight of the soul to the next world. Every window and door was flung open, all knots were unloosed and every mirror covered lest it should confuse the departing spirit. The soul was thought to linger in the house for a while, and candles were lit to ward off any malignant spirits which might threaten it. Watchers stayed by the body all night, and in some countries, notably Ireland, this practice developed into the wake at which merrymaking and feasting took place to give comfort to the soul before its journey into the unknown.

The fear of impeding the departure of the soul takes its most alarming form in the once-popular belief that one should never try to save a person from drowning. This idea was strengthened by the superstition that certain rivers claimed an annual toll of bodies. Some required only one, like the Dart in Devon and the Tweed, but others, like the Trent, demanded three. Should the river be cheated of its due it would quickly claim whoever had cheated it. There was the same superstition about the sea, which once made seamen reluctant to help a drowning colleague. It also accounts for the refusal of many of the older breed of sailors to learn to swim, for once the sea had decided to claim you, any attempt at escape was fruitless and merely prolonged the agony of drowning.

The belief that rivers demanded an annual human sacrifice was a relic of the ancient and powerful cult of river worship. The river made the land bordering it fertile; it supplied water for man and beast, and provided food in the fish that lived in it. But occasionally it would show its displeasure by flooding and destroying crops and life, and could only be placated by gifts or sacrifice. The sea, too, could be benign or cruel and great care was needed in handling corpses washed up on the shore. In primitive coastal communities it was thought dangerous to deprive the sea of its victim, and the body was hurriedly buried on the seashore between the high and low watermarks. In Christian countries it was thought that the sea could be placated only if the corpse were given a proper churchyard burial, but this was often opposed by the parish authorities because of the cost. In England it did not become a legal responsibility of the parish until 1808.

It was not the same if the victim drowned in a river. The object in such cases was the rapid recovery and burial of the body. It was commonly believed that the corpse rose to the surface on between the seventh and ninth day after drowning, and should it not do so many devices were used to locate it. Very common was the idea that a scooped-out loaf of bread carrying a small quantity of mercury, would float to where the body was and remain over it, an expedient used as recently as 1935 when a child was drowned in the Bridgwater Canal at Sale, Cheshire. The firing of a gun on the river bank was also thought to make the body float to the surface, and around the coast of Cornwall fisherman believed that their boat would come to a standstill when near a floating corpse.

Both the laying out of the body and the funeral was steeped in superstition in almost every country. The eyes of the dead person must be closed immediately, as the soul is thought to be seeking a companion on the journey soon to come. In some countries the clothes in which the corpse is buried must be unworn, and in the north of England a complete outfit ready for burial used to be collected and kept side-by-side with the wedding trousseau in the bottom drawer.

The ancient idea of disease-transference is met again if cancer was thought to be the cause of death. Butter was left overnight on the coffin in the belief that the cancer would leave the body and enter the butter, which was then thrown away. No doubt this custom resulted from the childlike belief that we shall all arise with our bodies complete on Judgement Day and that nothing must be allowed to interfere with this. The same reasoning is found in the burial with the body of amputated limbs. During the eighteenth century some people even insisted on being buried upside-down on the theory that, as the world would be upturned by the Last Trumpet, they would then be the right way up!

Help in seeing that the body would look respectable when the time came was extended more to women than to men, and in Scandinavia a mirror was always placed in the coffin for this purpose. The most important thing, however, in facing the hereafter, was to survive the rigorous questioning from St. Peter before final allocation could be made. The deceased had to show some proof of his goodness on earth. In many parts of England and America, well into the eighteenth century, it was customary to bury the corpse with Sunday School attendance certificates, while in Russia the coffin often contained a fulsome testimonial of the departed's conduct on earth provided by the village priest or elder.

Touching the corpse in the coffin, or merely looking at it, was thought to help dispel evil spirits and bring good fortune to the living. In many rural areas until quite recently it was the practice to invite friends in to touch the body before the coffin was closed, and the invitation was often extended to passing strangers. It would have been churlish and bad-mannered in the extreme to decline the invitation.

The funeral walk to the cemetery also had its traditions. A cure for warts was to touch them against the wood of the coffin, and the use of the metal coffin-handles as a cure for rheumatism and gout has already been mentioned. Rain on the coffin was a sure sign that the soul of the departed was at rest, but a shaft of sunlight falling on the face of a mourner meant that he would be the next to die.

The most serious danger to the soul was if the corpse were to be the first one buried in a new graveyard. The disturbed earth-spirits would inevitably demand a victim in compensation, and what better than the recently-liberated soul of the deceased, probably earth-bound until the funeral was over? This idea was hardly in keeping with orthodox Christian belief and was severely discouraged by most clergymen. Yet it persisted, and ingenious methods were devised to deal with the problem. Many an incumbent, carrying out the first burial in a new graveyard with no notable nervousness among the congregation, may well have congratulated himself on the ending of such pagan superstitions. He was probably unaware that he was holding not the first, but the second burial on the site, the first having been carried out in secret some time earlier with the corpse of a cat or dog. There is another deep-rooted belief that the soul of the last person buried must remain on watch in the graveyard until such time as a new arrival relieves him of his duties.

A curious legal superstition can still cause trouble even today. This is the belief that the passage of a coffin over private land creates a new right-of-way. This is quite untrue. But often an unseemly brawl broke out during a decorous journey to the church, if the funeral party took a short cut across a farmer's field. This is probably a relic of ancient Roman law, which held that if a man bought land which included graves, he must give access at all times to those wishing to visit them.

Two types of corpse stood little chance of burial in consecrated ground: suicides, and felons who had been hanged on the gallows. Suicides (and witches) were normally buried at cross-roads, and the last such burial took place in England in 1823 at the cross-roads at St. John's Wood, London, just outside what is now Lord's Cricket Ground. The bodies of those hanged on the gallows were usually exhibited on a gibbet, as a warning to others, until only the skeleton remained. The bones of such corpses were valued for their curative powers, and skulls were in great demand. A favourite Tudor cure for epilepsy was to drink from the skull of a hanged man. But the strangest of all cures was the hand of one who had been hanged—either a suicide or from the gallows. Its contact was said to cure at once goitre, tumours, cancer and sores of all kinds. Bodies hanging on the gibbet were often mutilated and the hands cut off for this purpose. The hand of a hanged felon could also be put to more sinister use. As the "Hand of Glory" it was well known throughout Europe and elsewhere as a charm to induce deep sleep and therefore as a useful aid to thieves and burglars. For this purpose the hand was pickled in brine, dried until iron-hard, and then used as a base for a candle made of the dead man's fat or that of a young girl. Such a candle, if lit in a house of sleeping people, would keep them snoring until the candle was put out—which could only be done by dousing it with milk. In some versions of this legend the fingers of the hand itself were lit as candles, and those which refused to light showed how many people were still awake in the house. The last known use of this odd device was in Ireland in 1832, where it proved a signal failure, as the would-be burglar fell over a bucket and roused the entire family.

Many variations are found on the Hand of Glory idea. In Czechoslovakia a human bone was used as a charm against waking, while in Hungary a leg bone was hollowed out to make a flute, whose music was claimed to induce instant and trance-like sleep in those who heard it. In India ashes from a funeral pyre were used to induce sleep and aid burglarious entry, while across the world in Mexico the forearm of a woman who had died in childbirth was used for a similar purpose. The principle was not always invoked for criminal reasons, and in Bulgaria the soil from a grave was often collected by young men who threw it over the house of the beloved in the hope the sleeping parents would stay asleep and not disturb their love-making.

Anything closely associated with a hanged man was valued, and nothing more so than the gallows rope. As late as 1940 in Scotland a strand from one was recorded as being used to cure epilepsy. The idea that the characteristics a dead person displayed in life could influence future events is found in several countries. In Russia, at times of drought, villagers would disinter the corpse of a person who had died from over-drinking in the hope that his capacity to attract liquid would precipitate a fall of rain. In the same way, aborigines exhume the bodies of twins if the crops fail, hoping that by showing them to the elements it would help double the crop.

There are many stories concerned with lights, and the dead or dying. A common belief is that if a small ball of light is seen in a churchyard it will finally move away and travel to the house of a person who is soon to die. Mysterious flames and fires rising over warriors' burial mounds are a regular feature of Icelandic sagas. The flames are thought to be the souls of the departed guarding their bodies.

There are persistent rumours that at the time of death a blue light is seen floating just above the dying person, and residents of Eastbourne, on the Sussex coast, claim to this day that at the time of the first Crumbles murder in 1920 mysterious "corpse lights" were seen hovering on the beach at the spot where the body of Irene Munro was later found buried.

The custom of lighting candles around a coffin was originally intended to drive away the evil spirits seeking the soul, and many are the beliefs connected with them. If a candle near a coffin were to blow out, severe illness or even death would overtake the person who had lit it. If the candle was on the altar before which a coffin lay, then the clergymen officiating at the funeral would not be long for this world. To leave a coffin in a house without lights was especially dangerous for the soul of the departed, and to leave the body in darkness and alone in a locked house was in effect to wish the dead person in Hell. According to E. and M. Radford's *Encyclopaedia of Superstitions*, an incident of this kind caused a bitter quarrel between neighbours on a modern housing estate as late as 1951.

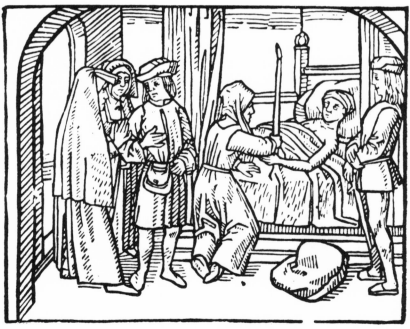

13 A candle for the evil spirits

Almost every culture has displayed, from its customs and beliefs, a real fear of the spirits of the departed. In civilized societies this fear is felt mainly in connection with earth-bound spirits. It is thought that they linger on earth perhaps to expiate some offence, and manifest themselves as apparitions haunting the place where murder was done or violent death took place. At Bisham Abbey, on the River Thames near Marlow, the ghost of an Elizabethan lady is still said to be seen wringing her hands in anguish near the spot where she murdered her backward child. Rumour, always wise after the event, insists that during repairs to the house some years later the skeleton of a small boy was indeed found there, still clutching the little slate upon which he was scratching his pitiful lessons. Yet only a few hundred yards away, along the river bank towards Marlow Bridge, is the waterside grave of Edith Rosse, thought by some to have been poisoned with arsenic in the 1920s and purposely buried there by Maundy Gregory so that all traces of poison would soon be washed away. So far no spectral socialite of the time has been seen to haunt the spot, nor have any manifestations been noted near Maundy Gregory's own grave in France. Poltergeists, who act in such a strange and erratic manner from time to time, are sometimes said to be the earth-bound spirits of the young wishing to stay in the company of children.

In more primitive communities the fear of the spirits of the dead is far more general. Fear of the dead may be associated with the personal name of the deceased, and no other member of the family is ever given the same name, for this is inviting the dead person to claim his kin for his own as soon as possible. Anyone who already has the same name as the dead person will hurry to change it, a custom which greatly confuses those studying the habits and customs of such tribes. North American Indians and Eskimos attach great importance to their name, believing it to be as much part of them as their eyes or teeth. Some consider that a name never dies, and, when old age approaches, they change their name to try to lengthen life. Intimate association with a personal name can make the owner refuse to divulge it or let it be spoken by any other person, in case he or she should acquire part of his soul. Though given a proper name at birth some Australian aborigines never allow it to be used, but are known by another name, such as that of a bird or animal.

This curious belief can be traced as far back as the ancient Egyptians, who, at birth, were given two names, the good name and the true name. The good name was in everyday use, and the true name carefully concealed. In some cultures a man may never mention his own name, though others may. Among the Indians of British Columbia no man would admit to his name, though he would willingly reveal the true name of other members of his community. They are not alone in this custom, and in Malaya husband and wife are never called by their own names but are described as "the father or mother" of their child, whose own name may be mentioned. The child, on the other hand, must never be called by his own name but is known as the child of so-and-so.

Further complications arise amongst the Kaffirs, where a man normally takes the name of an animal for his second title. But the spirit of the animal is "jealous" of this, and so speaking its name is taboo. Reference to the animal, and so to the man, must be oblique and descriptive, and in extreme cases must not even include similar-sounding words to the original. The Dyaks of Borneo believe that to mention the name of one's mother-in-law will incur the wrath of the Gods.

Fear of the spirits of the dead is world-wide, a fact noted by the Elizabethan colonists of Virginia more than three centuries ago. There they found the belief widespread that death held a list of names of the living and carried them off one by one. To circumvent this, when an Indian died, every other member of the community changed his name, so that Death would be confused and unable to identify the next victim.

Customs like these can create problems for anthropologists trying to trace a community's history. It is really difficult in the presence of customs, from California to South Australia, where it is forbidden to mention the name, or supply any information at all, about the dead. The ban may be limited only to the period of mourning, but sometimes it is permanent.

In some communities, even when fear of the dead does not reach these extremes, there exists a whole ritual of behaviour designed to preserve the memory of those departed. Many oriental peoples believe that ancestors' spirits dwell in certain trees. In China the family will plant a tree on the grave, in which the spirit may dwell; the evergreen cypress and pine are often planted, to bring strength and long life. In other communities a sacred tree stands at the entrance to each village, which is believed to contain the spirits of the dead. Such trees must never be cut or felled, or the aggrieved spirits will bring sickness on the villagers. These trees are sacred, and anyone passing them must honour their ancestors by bowing low to each tree. Certain African tribes have similar beliefs. Indeed, the situation can become awkward if the tree is valuable and represents a potential source of revenue. In such cases the ancestor-spirit must be induced to leave the tree, by spilling a little palm oil on the ground nearby. The spirit will leave the tree to sample the delicacy, and during its absence the tree can be felled. No one seems to worry that the unhoused spirit will be angry; it is just assumed that it will seek alternative accommodation in another tree. In other parts of Africa the same ruse is adopted, but a little house is built containing rice to tempt the spirit.

Perhaps one of the oddest beliefs connected with the dead is that the sins of the dead person can be transferred to somebody living who is willing to accept them. This idea harks back to the ancient belief in the scapegoat as a recipient of guilt or bad behaviour. In Britain the form of transfer usually consisted of eating food in the presence of the corpse, during a complicated ritual involving lighted candles. "Sin-eating" was common in the seventeenth century, and though stated by John Aubrey to be on the wane in his day, persisted in Wales and the Marches well into Victorian times. Some poor people in various villages actually became professional sin-eaters, performing this gruesome function either for payment, or for the food and drink which the ceremony involved. The amount of food varied; sometimes a mere crust of bread was placed on the corpse's breast and dutifully eaten by the volunteer. Sometimes a complete meal, including wine, was provided. Another common practice was to ask the sin-eater to eat some salt and drink some wine. Every drop of wine swallowed was thought to represent one sin the deceased had committed during his life. Many corpses would have been shocked to see the magnitude of their transgressions!

In other parts of England, notably in East Anglia, the custom persisted in living memory of putting a loaf and some salt on the coffin. A passing stranger was offered a little food, and ate it, unaware that he had acquired an extra burden of sin. For this reason, in this part of the country, the older countryfolk still have a reluctance to go anywhere near a house in which a death has taken place or where there might be a body.

Modern spiritualists, of course, have no part in such odd customs and superstitions. Yet they are rare in being one of the few groups who set out to make contact with the spirits of the dead. Through their efforts they hope to find out what lies beyond the grave, a problem that has exercised the minds of the most eminent thinkers of every age. That the grave is not the end is accepted by most civilizations. But real and certain knowledge of what may happen afterward still eludes us.

Our reluctance to accept the inevitability of death has resulted in a form of corpse-preservation which harks back 3,000 years to the ancient Egyptians. Embalming has long been popular in the United States of America, as it was in Egypt, but new techniques are now being applied based on the even more bizarre concept that the dead may one day be brought to life again. The technique used is that of cryogenics—deep-freezing so that the body does not decay but remains as it was in life. Thus, if a cure is one day found for the disease that ended life, the body may be restored from what is evidently considered a cataleptic state and the new treatment applied to it.

Parallel with this are the rather more realistic studies of ways of slowing down the ageing process. New medicines and new treatments are in any case tending to produce a longer expectation of life, with a corresponding increase in world population and a higher proportion of old people. Experiments with animals and fish suggest possible ways of extending life span apart from retarding disease. The temporary underfeeding of young rats early in life appears to slow their growth and, even when normal feeding is resumed, to slow their rate of ageing so much that some have lived twice as long as ordinary rats.

So with fish: the cooling of their environment results in slower growth and longer life, as does castration before sex organs have developed fully. A colder environment, however, has the opposite effect on warm-blooded animals. Again, the action of certain vitamins, notably C and E, has been shown to prolong the life of mice by inhibiting the ageing process of the chromosomes. Unfortunately there is no evidence that they do the same for human beings.

More relevant to human life span has been the study of exercise and its effect on preserving health and retarding the normal symptoms of old age. Recent findings seem to show that those who enjoyed moderate sport and exercise at college or university are likely to live longer than major athletes, or those who indulged in no athletics at all.

In view of the world's population crisis there are some who want an embargo on all experiments designed to prolong life. This is certainly not the accepted view in Britain, where in 1972 fifty doctors signed a letter to the *Lancet* calling for such experiments to continue. Much discussion has also taken place on the ethics of euthanasia, and a distinction has been drawn between negative euthanasia (the withholding of treatment that may prolong life) and positive euthanasia (the giving of treatment that may accelerate death). Opinion in the medical profession seems to be hardening in favour of negative euthanasia, and a recent American survey shows 60 per cent of hospital physicians to be in favour of it.

13

The Survival of
Superstition

MUCH of the medical folklore dealt with in these pages comes from primitive communities or from civilizations of the past. But a great deal of it remains alive today, not only in rural communities where new ideas permeate slowly, but among young people in cities and urban housing estates where they enjoy daily contact with the wonders of science.

It might seem something of a paradox that in today's sophisticated society superstition flourishes as much as ever. Many of the old beliefs have died, it is true: few people today really believe that sickness can be transferred to an inanimate object or to an animal to effect a cure. But other beliefs have arisen in their place, often due to an incomplete understanding of modern medical thought. Science and research are moving so fast, in fact, that often only the specialist is capable of understanding what is happening, and specialists are notorious for their inability to explain their findings to the layman. Only vaguely aware of their implications, the ordinary man retreats to the safety of superstition and magic. It is the sometimes unbelieveable implications of scientific discovery and research that convince him that there might be something in the old superstitions after all. He is forced to the conclusion that just because something cannot be explained, it may yet be true. It has been shown time and time again that research, particularly in medicine, vindicates beliefs that have been held for centuries. The folk cure of today may well become the medical sensation of tomorrow.

A secondary reason for the strength of supersition is the current disillusion with orthodox religion. Millions today have no hard religious convictions: there is nothing to stop them investigating the unknown. The simple faith of their ancestors, however comforting it may appear, seems just a symptom of blind belief and an un-enquiring mind. The resultant paradox is seen in many facets of life. Progressive thinkers, slowly stepping forward on the shifting sands of uncertainty, are only too glad to find a solid rock of belief beneath their feet even if that rock is merely an outcrop of what has gone before. A new image is given to old beliefs, and ideas that have existed for generations are proudly hailed as new thinking. Thus we see the revival of interest in herbal cures which are thousands of years old, and over-simplified religious cults such as the "Back to Jesus Movement." The sudden rise in interest in astrology and the occult is a sign of the search for some substitute for the old religions and a need to replace the comfort and assurance which they once supplied. The hundreds of horoscopes which appear in newspapers and magazines are avidly read by an estimated 80 per cent of the public, of whom some 20 per cent believe them to be true.

Modern techniques are applied to ancient beliefs and cults. The modern palmist, for example, no longer looks at the hand itself to foretell the future. He obtains a print of the palm which he studies at leisure, measuring the lines with care and exactitude. Spectacles of specially-ground and tinted lenses are made, which are claimed to help one perceive the "aura" of a person, though to what end is doubtful. The first British astrological shop was opened in London in 1973. Here one can buy crystal balls, divining rods, aids to palmistry, Tarot cards and the whole mumbo-jumbo of paranormal investigation and experiment. One notes that it is run by a well-known actor who, on his own admission, is one of the most superstitious members of a highly superstitious calling. Another actress has even evolved a method of foretelling the future and assessing one's health by closely examining the sole of the foot.

In medical superstitions, faith plays a large part, as is shown by the use of placebos in clinical trials. But there is enough solid evidence, even if unexplained, to justify the existence of many medical beliefs. Indeed, research is constantly revealing evidence of the truth of many long-held ideas, some of them so commonplace that one wonders why they needed investigating. In 1972 six American doctors published their findings on how newborn babies reacted when deprived of their mother's care during the first few days of birth. The study was concerned mainly with premature births, where this situation usually arises, but their findings merely confirmed what every mother has known from the beginning of time : that the effect of early mothering (called "extended contact" for the purpose of the trial) results in a happier and more contented baby.

Not that the study of medical folklore is always a waste of time. Doctors in Mexico have been studying the effect of the world-wide superstition that it is unlucky to cut a baby's nails, held in Latin-America to cause blindness or to make the child stutter. The result is that Mexican mothers provide their infants with mittens to stop them scratching with their long or rough nails. Several cases have come to light where a thread, being detached from the mitten and winding itself tightly around the infant's finger, has caused gangrene and, in two cases, necessitated amputation. Other beliefs are not so readily exploded. In England attention has been given to the widely-held theory that headaches are often a symptom of high blood pressure. More than four hundred headache victims were questioned and their blood pressures noted by a team from the Medical Research Council. They found no connection at all between headaches and blood pressure. Headaches do not imply raised blood pressure, and blood pressure does not always induce headaches. The same team also examined some of the fallacies about migraine, notably that intelligent people are more prone to this affliction. Once again the myth was exploded, and migraine shown to be just as prevalent among those of lower mentality. Neither of these findings was agreed with much enthusiasm by the public, and patients with chronic headache will continue to think their doctor neglectful if he does not test their blood pressure at the first opportunity. Doctors who have had long experience as family physicians often pander to their patients' wishes in such cases. They know how important it is to establish confidence, despite their private feelings about the value of the treatment or diagnostic method. Yet occasionally they make it obvious that they do not condone certain practices, as is seen in the differing attitudes about circumcision. Writing in *World Medicine* (1972) an American mother living in England told how appalled she was at the thinly-veiled hostility she met from English doctors and nurses when she enquired about circumcision for her newborn child. At present circumcision is performed as a routine at birth in America (as it was in this country fifty years ago) but fashions have changed. "Medical opinion in Britain is generally against it," she was severely told by her G.P. When asking advice from an independent medical authority she was given no definite advice for or against the operation, but was reminded, rather pointedly, that it was "a mutilating operation."

Circumcision was once routine in Britain, but modern thought is against it, despite theories linking uncircumcised males with cervical cancer in women. At present the subject is being investigated by the World Health Organisation, whose findings will no doubt decide whether circumcision is advisable or not. In the meantime information is lacking and the situation confused. Prejudice is rampant, and it is unfortunate that experienced physicians in civilized countries should have such divergent attitudes to such a simple medical matter. The situation is not uncommon. One of the more depressing aspects of reading the medical press regularly is to realize that doctors still cannot agree how to treat ailments which the ordinary man thinks were known generations ago. More than he realizes, the average patient is still very much a guinea pig.

There is less divergence of opinion about that other favourite operation of childhood—tonsillectomy. Most doctors are frankly against it and view the operation as needlessly exposing the child to discomfort and danger. They point out that about three children in 100,000 die as a result of the operation, while none have ever died from tonsilitis itself. The physical and mental shock to the child can be damaging: the child usually feels quite well on entering hospital and comes home feeling sick. Yet thousands of parents still insist on the operation, believing that it will alleviate the discomfort of sore throat and catarrh and will improve the general state of health of the child in later years.

In Britain some 200,000 tonsillectomies are performed every year, representing about a third of all admissions to hospital of children under the age of seven. There are even some parents who think that tonsils should be removed as a matter of routine, even if no trouble with the nose or throat is experienced. Doctors regard this devotion to tonsillectomy as a superstition which harks back to the old methods of bleeding and cupping. But superstitions die hard, and the incidence of demands for the operation is dropping only slowly by about 10 per cent a year.

The widespread fear of sterility following mumps in men has also been proved baseless. A team at a London hospital has published a study of nearly 200 men who had mumps in the five years before, and there was no evidence that the condition stopped them from fathering children. Men are highly sensitive to anything they think might affect their virility, a fact which often accounts for their doubts concerning vasectomy. In this operation a small incision is made which cuts the vas, the tiny tube which injects fertile sperm into the semen, while still allowing normal intercourse. Many men believe that enjoyment of the act will be reduced and their virility diminished; but there is no evidence to support this. Others fear that as the operation is irreversible it may create emotional problems if they marry for a second time and the new partner desires children. Some wives are unwilling to let their husbands undergo an operation which might remove one deterrent to extra-marital intercourse—the fear of pregnancy. This last is an important factor, for no operation for vasectomy on a husband can be undertaken without his wife's consent. Such doubts as these may be removed in the future by a new technique. The vas is cut, as before, but the two ends are no longer tied and sealed off. They are reconnected by a tiny plastic tube incorporating an on-off tap, which is turned to the "off" position after the operation. At any time in the future the tap can be turned on again by minor surgery, and the effect reversed.

Fear and emotional problems also arise in transplantations, particularly in heart transplants. For the surgeon the heart is just one organ of the body, like the liver, kidneys or lungs. But, for the patient, anything concerning his heart is affected by emotional overtones that can seriously disturb him, and prevent his recovery. Psychiatrists feel that a major factor in inducing such disorders is a patient's sense of awe at having *his* heart operated upon, particularly if the heart is opened. The result is very often a period of mental instability, the patient denying vehemently that his heart had actually been opened.

Unable to cope with the reality of the situation, the patient may try and escape from it by temporary mental withdrawal.

There has been some criticism that surgeons do not take enough account of the fears of transplant patients, concerning themselves only with the technical success of the operation. But much thought has been given to behaviour and mental states in the treatment of other physical conditions. Fatness is now being treated by behavioural therapy in which the patient is forced to study carefully almost every mouthful of every meal, to note not only what he eats, but how and when he eats, and learns to trace a pattern between his eating habits and, for example, anger or tiredness. Concentration on the subject of eating is said to result in a reduction in weight, though of course this may well be brought about by the patient's realization that he is eating too much and too often, and a reduced intake of food will therefore result. A more dangerous form of behavioural therapy is aversion therapy, at least when used in the treatment of what was once called the criminally insane. Two state institutions in California have been using a particularly barbarous form of aversion therapy on men with violent records, or who constantly attempted to mutilate themselves. Injections of the muscle-relaxing drug succinylcholine have been used, the effect of which is to create a feeling of asphyxiation with the certainty that death is near. General paralysis with almost complete inability to breathe prevails for about two minutes, during which time the prisoner is told that his condition is due to his bad conduct and will only improve if he behaves better in future. Such treatment is on a par with the eighteenth-century attitude to madmen who were placed in a spinning chair until they were almost insensible, and told that it was the result of their eccentric behaviour. What is even worse in the American cases is that treatment was given in contravention of the Nuremberg Code, devised after the World War Two trial of war criminals, and the Declaration of Helsinki—both of which lay down that experiments on human beings can be carried out only with their consent or with consent from their legal representative. Despite claims that the treatment with succinylcholine was not experimental, just a standard adjunct to shock treatment, both Californian institutions have stopped using this form of therapy.

On a more acceptable level, aversion therapy is often used in cures for smoking. Usually this takes the form of tablets of a metal salt, which, when swallowed before smoking, react with the nicotine to create a bad taste in the mouth. Gradually the body comes to link the bad taste with the cigarette, and smoking is reduced. Most doctors now have given up smoking, usually more by self-discipline than by such aversion techniques, and, oddly enough, are better at it than psychiatrists. Tests carried out on both types of practitioner in London and the Home Counties showed that 70 per cent of medical men gave up smoking purely by will power, but only 40 per cent of psychiatrists. The comment of a suburban tobacconist, asked his views on the warning notices printed on cigarette packets, was: "It'll scare them stiff, and everyone knows you smoke more when you're scared!"

Doctors and psychiatrists alike continue to delve into the beliefs and superstitions of the long-suffering public. One doctor has recently fulminated against the harmless belief that the provision of school milk is beneficial. The very few children who come to school hungry, says he, need a good meal and not just milk. Most of the others are fat, pale and constipated, and already suffering from the over-effects of milky and sugary foodstuffs. Dietary customs are a rich source of investigation. Studies have even been made of the strange habit of the Japanese to eat tangerines between meals, while travelling, in front of the television, and indeed at any time. Cases have been found of young children eating as many as 100 tangerines a day, resulting in the deposit of the pigment carotene on the palms of their hands and the soles of their feet, giving them a rich sunset-yellow colour, which was liable to be diagnosed as jaundice. One may wonder how yellowing of the skin in Japanese people is diagnosed at all, but the case is fully reported in the Journal of the American Medical Association. From Australia comes another report concerning the classic custom of using Worcester sauce as a reviver "the morning after." It seems it is a highly dangerous procedure, though it has apparently restored the flagging spirits of generations of regular army officers in messes around the world, and still does so. Research on this subject in Australia was undertaken on several patients whose fondness for the sauce had almost overtaken their fondness for alcohol. One bearded resident of the outback drank it by the glass several times a day, and between times used it as a gin chaser. He was found to be suffering from severe kidney damage and high blood pressure.

But far less dangerous pastimes than drinking neat Worcester sauce are solemnly investigated to assess the value of old customs. The simple act of sneezing is not as innocent as it seems, for there may be an association between the tissues of the nose and the erectile mechanism of the penis. Investigation shows that sneezing is very likely to occur after intercourse, so that what the wife may think is an incipient cold in her partner may just be a sign of a full and happy love-life.

A previous chapter examined some of the fallacies and folklore surrounding sex, conception and abortion. In today's society, where such matters are discussed interminably, new superstitions come to light and show the appalling ignorance which still exist in matters or sex, even among those who pride themselves on their progressive outlook. Boys and girls who copulate seem to remain blissfully unaware of the biological result of such activities. Many young people believe that intercourse performed in a standing position will not result in pregnancy, an idea which is as untrue as it is uncomfortable.

Preoccupation with sex has resulted, inevitably, in many misconceptions. Yet studies of matters remote from sex seem to return inexorably to that subject, and confirm the Freudian theory that sex lurks behind nearly everything. Biologists investigating the perfume of flowers now think that certain scents are caused by the breakdown of chemicals which can have sex-arousing properties. The custom of giving a bunch of flowers to the beloved may therefore have dark undertones and bouquets may soon feature as an artifact in sex-shops. Many of the sex "tonics" available in such places are based on the age-old theory of like-inducing-like. One of the newest forms of tonic is made from the velvet skin scraped from the antlers of the New Zealand deer, an animal famed for his unflagging sexual appetite. Once again we are back to old beliefs, derided not so long ago, but revived again and used as a bait for those who know nothing of history and must therefore pay to learn.

The use of medical superstition as a means of promoting sales is found even among the most ethical of pharmaceutical manufacturers. The Wellcome Foundation Ltd., associated with the Wellcome Trust, has access to the finest medical museum and library in the world, and points a contrast in its publicity between medical methods of a bygone age and the treatment now available. Far less reputable firms have used similar tactics, and one well-known brand of cold cure makes use of the common belief that an ordinary cold goes round the house for weeks in advertising the speed and success of its own product. Other companies in the patent medicine field point out that their products were popular in Victorian or Regency times as household cures. This particular form of publicity was for many years suspect in the world of advertising, where it was felt that a traditional image for a company might imply that it was rigid in its ways and unable to move with the times. But as today's fashion is interest in matters Victorian and Edwardian, a Victorian or Edwardian cough mixture should make the most of its ancestry.

Normally no publicity is needed to preserve the life of a medical belief. However outrageous it may seem, somebody, somewhere, still believes in it, and probably with good reason. Madness was once thought to be affected by the moon, and to be at its height when the moon was full. The very word lunatic derives from this superstition. Now it looks as if superstition might be the wrong word, for the American F.B.I. seems to have found a link between murders and the phases of the moon. Statistics kept over the last few years show a clear pattern of maximum murders at the full moon, though whether this is a pathological matter or associated with increased visibility at such times is a matter for conjecture. Many doctors believe that if the moon is strong enough to create tides and move millions of tons of water, then it might easily have a similar effect on body fluids, for example in the flow of blood across the brain.

Women are often said to be more superstitious than men, especially in medical matters. Certainly they have more reason to be. The start of the menstrual flow in childhood, the problems of conception and pregnancy, and the final and often extended phase of the menopause are all conditions which women must suffer in addition to normal illnesses.

Young girls experiencing their first period are naturally anxious at what seems an inordinate quantity of blood. Far too often no prior warning has been given by the mother, who assumes, often quite wrongly, that her daughter has already discussed it with friends. This may be so, but does not mean that she really understands what is happening, even if she has been expecting it. A common belief among girls, which often extends into later life, is that the menstrual flow represents the elimination from the body of something unhealthy or unclean. It is, of course, a perfectly normal and healthy process in which the lining of the womb, ready to nourish the egg cell produced each month, is automatically renewed if the egg remains unfertilized fourteen days later. The very nature of the womb lining that is being discarded can cause alarm initially, for unlike normal blood it does not usually clot, and once reaching the outside of the body can emit a pungent and unpleasant odour. Yet at the same time the average amount of blood produced at a monthly period is rather less than two fluid ounces, a fact which many women seem unable to believe. Ideally the event should be painless, but where a pregnancy has never been established the womb is likely to become cramped and irritated, resulting in the familiar period pain. Menstruation is stimulated by various hormonal substances produced by different glands in a delicate and complex process which naturally affects the well-being of the subject. Young girls may experience hot or cold flushes at such times and other transitory symptoms which, if unexplained, can create alarm and depression. More than one young girl has been driven to deep despair by being told that hot flushes were the sign of a guilty conscience.

Numerous are the ideas to which many women still cling surrounding the menopause, or change of life, when the monthly periods cease. The ending of a bodily function which has been going on more or less regularly for thirty years or more cannot be faced without some disturbance; only about 15 per cent of women suffer no symptoms during this period. The rest experience conditions ranging from hot flushes (by far the most common symptom) to headaches, giddiness, nervous instability and rheumatic pains, while more than a third begin to put on weight. The incidence of these disorders is not greatly different in the married or the unmarried, nor among those who have borne children and those who have not. Virtually the only noticeable difference is that the married woman who has had children is more likely to put on weight than the unmarried woman.

The changes of body function experienced by women at middle age often coincide with external symptoms. The skin becomes wrinkled, and many women are alarmed at the sudden appearance of fine facial hairs. There are several superstitions associated with this, perhaps the strongest being that bad luck will follow any effort to fight it, and that cutting or shaving will make it grow thicker still.

One of the most persistent fallacies associated with the change of life is that a woman's sexual capacity comes to an end. This springs from the mistaken belief that to feel any sexual satisfaction the womb and ovaries must be functioning. Many elderly couples disprove this theory, but the fear in many women that the menopause may not only end their capacity for motherhood, but also reduce their value as a wife, often brings on a quite needless depression. Any woman anxious on this score can take comfort from the remark of Céleste Vénard, later la Comtesse de Chabrillan, a famous Parisian beauty of the nineteenth century. When asked, late in life, at what age sexual desire diminished she replied, "You must talk to someone older, for I am only seventy!"

The fear of the unknown exerts its influence as much today as it did in the past. It may result in such apparent anachronisms as the incident in Esher, Surrey, in 1972 when Mrs. Marie Cooper, a gipsy, put a curse on the Clerk to the District Council when he served an order on her family to vacate a field on which their caravan was parked. It is doubtful if the Clerk, or anyone else on the Council, really believed in the influence of the curse. Yet, strangely enough, alternative accommodation was quickly found and Mrs. Cooper obligingly lifted her malevolent spell.

In the field of medical research fear of the unknown is seen in its modern form in the immense precautions taken before a new drug or treatment is released to the public. Inevitably this slows the development of new products and can result in new techniques remaining in the category of folk medicine in the absence of satisfactory clinical trials and official acceptance. This has happened in Italy where, for nineteen years, Dr. Liberio Bonifacio campaigned for official recognition of his theory that a substance extracted from goat glands might be a cure for cancer.

In France another Italian, the electrical engineer and radar specialist, Antoine Priore, has built at Bordeaux a machine which he claims has inhibited the growth of cancerous tissue in rats by electro-magnetic radiation and cured sleeping-sickness in mice. Despite impressive evidence of the validity of this claim, and support from many scientists, the inventor refuses to disclose his technical data, and "L'Affaire Priore" continues to divide medical opinion. Through the French Government's "Délégation Générale" for Scientific Research, finance has been allocated for more experiments to be held to confirm what is agreed by many, that radiation does, in some unknown manner, stimulate the defence mechanism of the body. Many other experienced scientists insist that Priore, who has no medical qualifications, is hoodwinking the medical profession as surely as did Elisha Perkins with his Metallic Tractors in the early nineteenth century.

Situations like this stem from unbelief and ultra-caution rather than from superstition. But superstition can still be created as a spin-off from modern discoveries and techniques. In 1963 it was suddenly realized that some Indians in Peru were becoming unaccountably hostile to any white men who ventured into their territory or explored the river banks. Anglers were shot at, boating parties on the Amazon threatened and warned off by Indians who were not only aggressive but also obviously in a state of panic. It took some time for the Government to find out the reason for this. It turned out that a rumour had started in the jungle that *gringos* (Americans, English or any blond foreigners) were hunting down Indians and shooting them to melt down their bodies and extract the fat. This fat, the rumour insisted, was an essential ingredient in the manufacture of atomic weapons, and the United States had received huge contracts from other countries to supply it. Immediate action was taken by the U.S. Government to dispel these fears, and things very quickly returned to normal. Yet there was some justification for the fear of the Indians, if one looked at the history of Peru. In the sixteenth century the Spanish conquistadores had used animal fat to grease and polish their weapons. Rumour had it that sometimes they killed Indians for this purpose. The legend had lived on. This story was easily adapted to modern times and weapons, and revived a belief that had lain dormant for more than three centuries.

Mankind is largely ignorant, but long of memory. Superstition will continue to flourish in the wake of scientific progress. Perhaps it is just as well, if it acts as a safety-valve and an escape route from the full realization of what the future may hold.

BIBLIOGRAPHY

The author wishes to acknowledge his debt to the Folklore Society and to the Trustees of the Wellcome Historical Medical Museum and Library for the facilities provided for research. Acknowledgement is also made to the authors and publishers of the following works consulted.

BOOKS

Baumler, E. *In Search of the Magic Bullet*. London: Thames and Hudson, 1965.
Black, W. G. *Folk Medicine*. New York: Burt Franklin, 1883; 1970.
Change of Life, "Medica." Delisle Ltd., 1949.
Drake, Emma. *What a Young Wife Ought to Know*. Vir Publishing Company, 1900.
Ellis, E. S. *Ancient Anodynes*. London: William Heinemann Medical Books, 1946.
Franklyn, Julian. *Death by Enchantment*. New York: G. P. Putnam, 1971.
Fryer, P. *The Birth Controllers*. London: Martin Secker & Warburg, 1965.
Frazer, Sir James. *The Golden Bough*. New York: Macmillan, 1954.
Hole, Christina. *English Folklore*. London: B. T. Batsford, 1940.
Inglis, B. *Drugs, Doctors and Disease*. London: Mayflower Books, 1965.
Jacob, Dorothy. *Cures and Curses*. New York: Taplinger Publishing Company, 1967.
Jameson, E. *The Natural History of Quackery*. London: Michael Joseph, 1961.
Jarvis, D. *Folk Medicine: A Vermont Doctor's Guide to Good Health*. New York: Holt, Rinehart and Winston, 1958.
King, Maurice H., ed. *Medical Care in Developing Countries*. New York: Oxford University Press, 1966.
Kourennoff, Paul M. *Russian Folk Medicine*. London: Pan Books, 1970.
Mair, Lucy. *Witchcraft*. New York: McGraw-Hill, 1969.
Maple, Eric. *Medicine, Magic and Quackery*. London: Robert Hale, 1968.
—————. *Superstition and the Superstitious*. London: W. H. Allen, 1971.
Matthews, L. *History of Pharmacy in Britain*. College Park, Md.: McGrath, 1962.

Maxwell, Nicole. *The Jungle Search for Nature's Cures.* New York: Ace Books, 1961.

Palos, Stephen. *The Chinese Art of Healing.* New York: Bantam Books, 1972.

Pelligrew. *Superstition in Medicine and Surgery.* London: J. A. Churchill, 1844.

Petulengro, Leon. *The Roots of Health.* New York: New American Library, 1970.

Pollack and Underwood. *The Healers.* London: Thomas Nelson and Sons, 1968.

Radford, E. and M. *Encyclopedia of Superstitions.* Chester Springs, Pa.: Dufour Edition, 1969.

Rivers, W. *Medicine, Magic and Religion.* Finch, 1924.

Rosenburg, C. *The Cholera Years.* Chicago: University of Chicago Press, 1962.

Sitwell, Edith. *English Eccentrics.* New York: Vanguard Press, 1971.

Thomas, Mai. *Grannies Remedies.* London: Wolfe Publishing Ltd., 1965.

Thorwald, Jurgen. *Science and Secrets of Early Medicine: Egypt—Babylonia—India—China—Mexico—Peru.* New York: Harcourt Brace Jovanovich, 1963.

Turner, E. S. *Taking the Cure.* London: Michael Joseph, 1967.

Underwood, P. *Into the Occult.* New York: Drake, 1973.

Walker, Kenneth. *The Story of Medicine.* New York: Oxford University Press, 1955.

Walters, F. *Household Dictionary of Medicine.* Swan, Soonenschein Ltd., 1895.

Wannan, W. *Bill Wannan's Folk Medicine.* London: William Collins Sons, 1972.

Wellcome, Henry. *Ancient Cymric Medicine.* Wellcome Foundation Ltd., 1909.

————. *Medicine of Ancient Erin.* Wellcome Foundation Ltd., 1909.

Wesley, John. *Primitive Remedies.* (Originally published as *Primitive Physick.*) Los Angeles: Woodbridge Press, 1947: 1973.

White, T. H. *The Age of Scandal.* Baltimore: Penguin Books, Inc., 1962.

Wilson, Colin, and Pitman, P. *Encyclopedia of Murder.* London: Pan Books, 1961.

Without Prescription. OHE Publications, 1968.

Wood, Clive, and Suitters, Beryl. *The Fight for Acceptance.* Medical Technical Publications, 1970.

JOURNALS

British Medical Journal
Chemist and Druggist
Journal of the American Medical Association
Journal of the Folklore Society

Lancet
New England Journal of Medicine
Pharmaceutical Historian
Pharmaceutical Journal
Pharmacie Mondiale
Practitioner
Pulse
World Health Organization Newsletters
World Medicine

INDEX

A

Abortion, methods of, 41
Acupuncture, 141–2
Aesculapius, 16
Africa, 10, 23, 25, 34
Alcoholism, treatment of, 97–8, 124
Anaesthesia, 19, 149
Aninga plant, 26
Aphrodisiacs, 18, 30–31
Aphrodite, Temple of, 31
Astrological shop, 173
Astrology, 11, 16, 76–7
Atomic weapons, human fat for, 183
Australian aborigines, 11, 25, 122, 168
Aversion therapy, 177
Aztecs, 78

B

Babylon, 31
'Back to Nature' movement, 133–4
Bantu tribe, 12
Baptism, 50
Barber-surgeons, 76, 89
Barker, Sir Herbert, 102, 136
Barrenness, 25
Bath, 145
Beddoes, Dr. Thomas, 148
Beecham, Thomas, 66–7
Berkeley, Mrs. 104
Binggeli, Johannes (Forest Brotherhood), 113
Birth, circumstances of, 33
Birth Control movement, 47–8
Boots the Chemist, 44

Borneo, 25
Bradlaugh (Charles) and Besant (Annie), 47
Breasted, James (Egyptologist), 17
Brighton, 154
Brittany, 22
Buganda, 23
Burial customs, 164

C

Caesarian birth, 33
Candles round coffin, 166
Cantharides (Spanish Fly), 18, 30
Carbolic Smoke Ball Co., 68
Casanova, 44, 151
Cats, 50, 122–3
Caul as guard against drowning, 33
Celestial Bed, 28
Change of life (menopause), 181
Changelings, 50, 54
Charaka Samhita (Indian) 78
China, 10, 26
Chinese Academy of Traditional Medicine, 143
Chinese herbal remedies, 75, 87
Chiropractice, 137–8
Cholera epidemics, 109, 121
Christian Church (Early), 18, 105
Christian Science, 108
Coffins, 164, 166
Colonic irrigation, 26
'Compleat Housewife' (1753), 27, 51
Comstock, Anthony, 47
Condoms, 43–4
Confetti, 25

189

Seventh Day Adventists, 110
Sevigné, Madame de, 43, 151
Sex-act to encourage crops, 23–5
Sexual desire, 182
Shadow, 13
Shaman, 16
Shen-Nung (Emperor of China), 18
Siam, 10
Siberia, 16
Sin-eating, 169
Sioux Indians, 36
Sloane, Sir Hans, 135
Smedley's Hydro, Matlock, 149
Smith, Edwin (Egyptologist), 17
Sorcery, 10
Soul, loss of, 10, 14
Soul, release of, 161
South Pacific Islands, 14
Spanish Fly (cantharides), 18, 30
Spas in England and America, 146
Spas in Europe, 151
Stephens, Joanna, 93
Still, Andrew Taylor, 102, 136
Stopes, Dr. Marie, 47–8
Succession Powder, 130

T

Taboos, 10–12
Tacitus, 11
Tahiti, 34
Takeda Chemical Co (Kyoto), 87
Tangerines, excess of, 179
Teetotalism, origin of, 157
Temperance Movement, 155–9
'Theory of Internal Disease' (Chinese), 18
Total Abstinence movement, 156–7
Tractoration, 99
Tradescant, John, 77
Transference of disease, 51, 122–4, 162
Transplants, 176

Triplets, 23
Twins, 23

U

Umbilical cord, 55

V

V-sign (Churchillian), 129
Vasectomy, 176
Vespasian, Emperor, 11
Vichy (France), 145

W

'Wandering' womb, 41
Wedding-cake, 25
Weighing witches, 14, 15
Weissenberg, Joseph (Community of St. John), 113
Wellcome, Henry, 69–70
Wesley, John, 83–4, 117, 124, 147, 151
Wet-nurses, 57–8
Whippers, 104
Whooping-cough cures, 51, 122
Witch-craft murder (1945), 131
Witch-doctors, duties of, 11
Womb, 41, 181–2
Writers taking drugs, 119

Y

Yellow Emperor's Classic of Internal Medicine (Chinese), 49
Yin and Yang in Chinese medicine, 141
Yoga Research Centre, Hyderabad, 105

Z

Zoser, King of Egypt, 17
Zulus, 55